ACSM/NCHPAD Resources for the Certified Inclusive Fitness Trainer

First Edition

EDITOR
Cary Wing, Ed.D., FACSM

ACSM/NCHPAD RESOURCES FOR THE CERTIFIED INCLUSIVE FITNESS TRAINER

First Edition

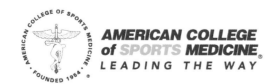

AMERICAN COLLEGE
of SPORTS MEDICINE®
LEADING THE WAY

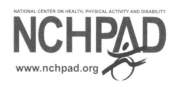

NATIONAL CENTER ON HEALTH, PHYSICAL ACTIVITY AND DISABILITY

NCHPAD

www.nchpad.org

American College of Sports Medicine, Indianapolis, IN
National Center on Health, Physical Activity and Disability, Birmingham, AL
Copyright © 2012 by the American College of Sports Medicine

Permissions Coordinator
American College of Sports Medicine
401 West Michigan Street, Indianapolis, IN
Indianapolis, IN 46202
www.acsm.org

Ordering Information:
Please contact the American College of Sports Medcine: Tel: (317) 637-9200; or visit www.acsm.org.

DISCLAMER
Care has been taken to confirm the accuracy of the information present and to describe generally accepted practices. However, the authors, editors, and publisher are not responsible for errors or omissions or for any consequences from application of the information in this book and make no warranty, expressed or implied, with respect to the currency, completeness, or accuracy of the contents of the publication. Application of this information in a particular situation remains the processional responsibility of the practitioner; the clinical treatments described and recommended may not be considered absolute and universal recommendations.

Printed in the United States of America

ISBN 978-1-885377-02-9
First Edition

GET ACSM CERTIFIED

You may be new to the field of sports medicine. Or maybe you're an experienced veteran in the profession. What matters most is that you've made the commitment to establish yourself as a reputable fitness professional. By working toward an American College of Sports Medicine Certification, you're on your way to earning one of the most highly recognized certifications in the industry.

CHOOSE A CERTIFICATION CATEGORY:

Health Fitness Certifications

Are you a fitness professional working in a health club or other community setting? Get certified and earn your ACSM Certified Group Exercise Instructor, ACSM Certified Personal Trainer, or ACSM Certified Health Fitness Specialist credential so you can work with healthy individuals or those with well-controlled health challenges.

Clinical Certifications

The ACSM Certified Clinical Exercise Specialist and ACSM Registered Clinical Exercise Physiologist credentials identify clinical professionals who are highly skilled in exercise management, testing, training and can also provide patients with therapeutic physical activity in a clinical setting.

Specialty Certifications

Do you already have an NCCA accredited certification? Add an ACSM specialty certification so you can work with special-needs clients. Currently there are three available, incuding: ACSM/ACS Certified Cancer Exercise Trainer; ACSM/NCHPAD Certified Inclusive Fitness Trainer (the subject of this resource manual); and ACSM/NPAS Physical Activity in Public Health Specialist.

The American College of Sports medicine, founded in 1954, is the world's largest sports medicine and exercise science organization with more than 50,000 national, regional, and international members and certified professionals in more than 90 countries. With professionals representing more than 70 occupations, ACSM offers a 360-degree view of sports medicine and exercise science. From academicians to students and from personal trainers to physicians, the association of public health, health/fitness, clinical exercise, and health care professionals is dedicated to helping people worldwide live longer, healthier lives through science, education, medicine, and policy. For more information, visit www.acsm.org, HYPERLINK "http://www.acsm.org/facebook" www.acsm.org/facebook, and HYPERLINK "http://www.twitter.com/acsmnews" www.twitter.com/acsmnews.

CONTRIBUTORS

Bobbi-Jo Atchison, B.P.E.

Donna Bernhardt Bainbridge, PT, Ed.D., ATC

Molly Blair, B.S., ACSM CIFT

Kathleen M. Cahill, M.S., ACSM RCEP

Brian J. Coyne, M.Ed., ACSM RCEP, ACSM CIFT

Yuri Feito, Ph.D., MPH, ACSM RCEP

Holly Giguere, B.S., CTRS, ACSM HFS

Jennifer N. Green, M.S.

Samantha Blythe Hiss, M.S., ACSM RCEP

Lamont Kelly

Carol Kutik, M.A., ACSM CIFT

Carolyn Lullo, M.S.

Chris Mackey, B.S.

Laurie A. Malone, Ph.D.

Jessica Malouf PT, DPT

Susan Ostertag, PT, DPT, NCS

James A. Peterson, Ph.D., FACSM

Karen Slater, M.A.

Jamie Terry, DPT, CSCS

Stephen J. Tharrett, M.S.

Meg Ann Traci, Ph.D.

Kirsti Van Dornick, BSc. Kin.

REVIEWERS

Andrew Mark Bosak, Ph.D., ACSM HFS, CSCS
Armstrong Atlantic State University

Richard Cotton, M.A., ACSM CES, ACSM PD
American College of Sports Medicine

Kim DeLeo B.S , ACSM CPT
Health and Exercise Connections, LLC

Sabrina Fairchild, M.A., ACSM HFS
California State University, Chico
Butte Community College

David G. Lorenzi, Ed.D., CAPE
Indiana University of Pennsylvania

Thomas Patrick Mahady, M.S., CSCS
Hackensack University Medical Center

Sharon Lynne McGoff, B.S., JD, ACSM HFS
Fit 4 Life Coaching, LLC

Ildiko Nyikos, M.A., ACSM RCEP
Founder, SeniorExerciseAtHome.com

Brooke Tafflinger, B.S., CTRS
Carmel Clay Parks and Recreation

Catherine Titus, M.Ed
Irvine Unified School District

Mark Zaleskiewicz, M.S., ACSM CES, FAACVPR
Shore Medical Center

PREFACE

The American College of Sports Medicine (ACSM) in collaboration with The National Center on Health, Physical Activity and Disability (NCHPAD) has developed a specialty certification for fitness professionals. Become an ACSM/NCHPAD Certified Inclusive Fitness Trainer and provide clients who are challenged by physical, sensory or cognitive disabilities with the appropriate knowledge and support to lead a healthy and comfortable lifestyle. To assist in obtaining the certification, ACSM and NCHPAD are proud to introduce the First Edition of the *ACSM/NCHPAD Resources for the Inclusive Fitness Trainer*. This manual is written by industry experts and is designed to provide guidance for fitness professionals who want to learn more about inclusive fitness and the pathway to certification.

It is estimated that 50 million people in this country have some type of disability, and they need health and fitness services. This significant portion of the population faces some of the greatest health risks associated with sedentary lifestyles. This population includes the young, adults, and seniors with physical, cognitive and/or sensory challenges—a wide range of individuals who must incorporate physical activity into their daily lives. There is a need for knowledgeable, certified trainers to deliver safe, relevant, and effective exercise programs to people with disabilities.

The *ACSM/NCHPAD Resources for the Inclusive Fitness Trainer* serves as a platform for fitness professionals to begin the process of learning about people with disabilities and learning how to develop an exercise prescription and program specifically for this population to become a Certified Inclusive Fitness Trainer (CIFT).

Before beginning to study the information in the manual, you should first read the Fact Sheet **"People First Language—Describing People with Disabilities,"** Appendix A. The information lays the groundwork to better understand people with disabilities and the educational material provided in the *ACSM/NCHPAD Resources for the Inclusive Fitness Trainer*.

Section I introduces fitness professionals to the field and profession of inclusive fitness training. A thorough review of the field is provided and this section identifies the need for certified trainers as well as opportunities for career development.

Of course, there needs to be a fundamental understanding of how the fitness industry reached this point. **Section II** explains the background and history of the Americans with Disabilities Act (ADA) with particular emphasis on promoting basic accessibility in health and fitness facilities.

Section III explains the screening process and the client consultation. The development of appropriate client-centered goals and objectives can only be achieved through a thorough risk assessment that includes physical fitness and functional testing. Knowing the red flags that are associated specifically with each client is essential for working with individuals with disabilities—as it is with all clients.

The next chapters in **Section IV** discuss exercise prescription and programming. To be successful as a fitness professional, the trainer needs to understand fundamental exercise program design considerations relating to flexibility and balance, resistance training, and cardiopulmonary training. This section provides information to design a safe, effective, and relevant exercise program for individuals with disabilities.

Section V is an overview of disability awareness relative to specific conditions such as spinal cord lesions, neuromuscular conditions, cognitive disorders, and non-progressive brain injuries. The fitness professional may find an individual has one or more of these conditions simultaneously and therefore need to understand the guidelines for managing each and every one.

The final chapter in Section VI addresses risk management and safety considerations. This information is standard in the fitness industry; however, the level of risk for a person with a disability can be even higher, depending on the circumstances—particularly, those situations that entail physical activity. As such, the primary key to dealing with risk is to anticipate it and have a specific plan for dealing with it, including doing whatever is reasonably possible to minimize the risk.

The goal of the *ACSM/NCHPAD Resources for the Inclusive Fitness Trainer* manual is to meet the needs of fitness professionals who want to develop an expertise in the area of inclusive fitness and become a certified trainer. We wish you success in achieving certification and empowering those who are challenged by physical, sensory or cognitive disabilities to live life to the fullest.

Cary H. Wing, Ed.D., FACSM
Editor

ACKNOWLEDGEMENTS

The editor would like to extend a special thanks to colleagues who so graciously provided peer reviews for this book and shared their expertise with me and the contributing authors: Jennifer Green; Blythe Hiss; Elizabeth Toumajian; Karen Slater; Suzanne Gray; Mike Heideman; Kerry Wiley; Janice Fitzgerald; and Donna Bainbridge. Finally I want to thank the American College of Sports Medicine (ACSM) and the National Center on Health, Physical Activity and Disability (NCHPAD) for their commitment and dedication to the industry.

Note: In August 2012 the 13-year-old National Center on Physical Activity and Disability (NCPAD) became the National Center on Health, Physical Activity and Disability (NCHPAD). Visit the website for more information: www.nchpad.org

This content was made possible in-part by support from the National Center on Health, Physical Activity, and Disability. NCHPAD is located in Birmingham, AL as part of the University of Alabama at Birmingham (UAB)/Lakeshore Research Collaborative. NCHPAD is supported by Grant/Cooperative Agreement Number U59DD000906 from the Centers for Disease Control and Prevention (CDC). The contents are solely the responsibility of the authors and do not necessarily represent the official views of CDC.

TABLE OF CONTENTS

Section IV Exercise Prescription & Programming

Section V Disability Awareness

Section VI Risk Management and Safety Considerations

Appendices

Index

Section I

Introduction to the Field
and Profession of
Inclusive Fitness Training

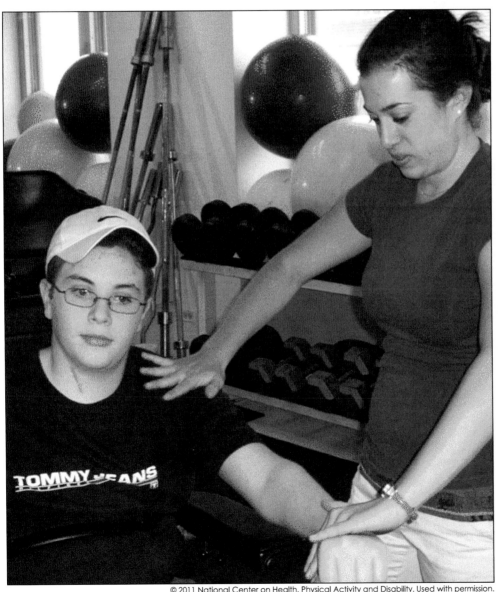

CHAPTER 1

Review of the Field and Profession of Personal Training

By Carolyn Lullo, M.S.

Carolyn Lullo, M.S., holds a bachelors degree from Miami University where she majored in Exercise Science and a masters degree from University of Illinois at Urbana-Champaign in Kinesiology. Upon completion of her masters degree, Carolyn worked as Assistant Director of Fitness at Miami University's Recreational Sports Center. She is currently completing her Ph.D. in Disability Studies at the University of Illinois at Chicago (UIC) and is focusing on health promotion/physical activity and disability. While at UIC she worked at the National Center on Health, Physical Activity and Disability and is now the AUCD/NCBDDD Fellow in Disability and Health Promotion.

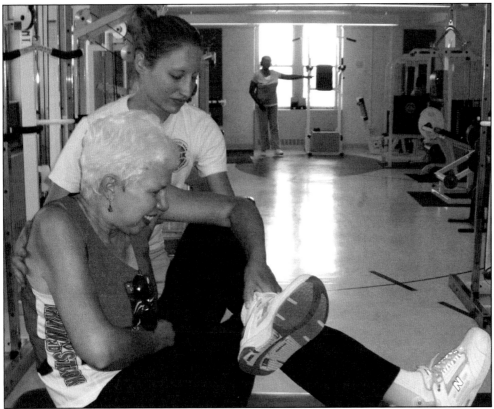

© 2011 National Center on Health, Physical Activity and Disability. Used with permission.

The Need for the Personal Training Profession

Over the past several years there has been increasing concern over the health of the U.S. population. In 2005, nearly 50% of the population had at least one chronic disease.[1] Chronic diseases include, for example, heart disease, arthritis, diabetes, and stroke and are largely preventable. Despite their preventable nature, the U.S. Centers for Disease Control and Prevention report that chronic diseases are the leading cause of death and disability in the U.S., accounting for 7 out of 10 deaths each year.[2,3] Of significant concern is the increasing number of individuals who are obese. Healthy People 2020 reports that only 30.8% of adults are at a healthy weight while 34.0% of adults and 16.2% of children and adolescents aged 2–19 years are considered obese.[4]

Physical activity is highlighted as a primary means of preventing chronic diseases and reducing obesity levels. In addition to reducing and preventing chronic diseases, physical activity improves weight status, reduces depressive symptoms, improves cardiorespiratory function and muscular fitness among many other benefits. [4]   Unfortunately, there is a general lack of adequate levels of physical activity throughout the population. In 2008, the U.S. Department of Health and Human Services published the *Physical Activity Guidelines for Americans*. These guidelines suggest that adults should engage in at least 150 minutes per week of moderate intensity or 75 minutes per week of vigorous intensity aerobic activity.[5] Evidence shows that more than 80% of adults and adolescents do not meet these minimum levels of physical activity.[4]

The low levels of physical activity are attributed to many variables, including not knowing how to exercise, not knowing where to exercise, sedentary occupations, lack of time, lack of motivation, and lack of opportunity.[4,6] The Inclusive Fitness Trainer is uniquely positioned to intervene upon many of these barriers to physical activity and thus increase physical activity levels resulting in decreased obesity levels and a reduction in the prevalence of chronic diseases. Research has shown that personal training can positively influence attitudes towards physical activity, lead to higher levels of attendance in physical activity sessions, and increase training load.[7,8,9] It can even lead to greater strength gains, greater improvements in VO_2max, and greater reductions in waist circumference and body fat when compared to individuals who did not receive personal training services.[9,10]

The Personal Trainer

The American College of Sports Medicine (ACSM) defines the Certified Personal Trainer (CPT) as, "a fitness professional who develops and implements an individualized approach to exercise leadership in healthy populations and/or those individuals with medical clearance to exercise."[11] According to ACSM, the CPT's scope of practice includes:

(1) Leading and demonstrating safe and effective methods of exercise by applying the fundamental principles of exercise science.

(2) Writing appropriate exercise recommendations.

(3) Motivating individuals to begin and to continue with their healthy behaviors.[11]

While an understanding of the science of exercise and how to safely implement an exercise program is important for the personal trainer, equally as important is an understanding of human interaction, individual barriers to physical activity, and motivational techniques that meet individual needs. In order to fulfill this scope of practice, personal trainers must be knowledgeable in: exercise prescription and programming; exercise physiology and related exercise science; health appraisal and fitness exercise testing; clinical and medical considerations; nutrition and weight management; safety, injury prevention, and emergency procedures; human behavior; and program administration, quality assurance, and outcome assessment.[11]

Education and Certification

Personal trainers most often receive their education in one or more of the following ways: college education, certification, on-the-job training, and professional experience. More and more frequently, colleges and universities are offering programs that prepare students for a career in the fitness industry. Individuals with an interest in personal training can pursue an education in majors such as kinesiology, exercise science, physical education, fitness specialist, and other related fields.

Even with a college degree, though, many employers still expect personal trainers to have an accredited certification before hiring.[12] There are a growing number of organizations that offer certifications, so it is important for the individual seeking certification to determine the level of recognition that a certification receives in the field and to investigate whether the certification is accredited by the National Commission for Certifying Agencies (NCCA).[13] In addition, requirements differ between employers. Therefore, it is important for the Inclusive Fitness Trainer to consult with facilities and programs that are similar to their desired place of employment and practice. Before pursuing any certification, potential personal trainers should determine if they meet the minimum eligibility requirements identified by the certifying organizations (figure 1.1).

Employment

Options for employment settings for personal trainers have expanded over the years. Health clubs continue to be the most popular setting, with approximately 61% of personal trainers working in this setting. [12] Health clubs, however, are quite varied in size, cost, and clients served. They can range from large, for-profit organizations to smaller, non-profit, community-based organizations. Corporate wellness centers and health clubs are growing in popularity as well. Medical fitness centers, which are a marriage between the healthcare field and fitness industry, offer another option for personal trainers. Ad-

---

Figure 1.1: What qualifications are necessary to become an ACSM/NCHPAD Certified Inclusive Fitness Trainer?

The ACSM Certification web site shares the following requirements must be met:
- Current ACSM Certification or a current NCCA-accredited, health/fitness-related certification (e.g., ACE, NCSF, NASM, NFPT, NSCA, Cooper Institute, etc.) OR
- Bachelor's degree in Exercise Science, Recreation Therapy, OR Adapted Physical Education AND
- Current Adult CPR (with practical skills component) & AED

---

ditionally, many personal trainers opt for the self-employment option, utilizing client's homes, public places, or studio spaces to conduct the exercise session.[14]

Personal training salaries vary greatly, depending on employment setting, employment status, education, and years of experience. The Bureau of Labor Statistics reports that the annual salary for "Fitness Trainers" ranges from $17,070 to $63,400, with a median salary of $31,090.[15] Hourly wages range from $8.21 to $30.48, with a median of $14.95.[15] According to a 2010 survey of 3,000 fitness professionals conducted by the American Council on Exercise (ACE), educational level is positively related to salary, but years of experience in the field plays an even more significant role.[16]

Code of Ethics

All American College of Sports Medicine Certified Professionals (ACSMCPs), are expected to work within the bounds of the Code of Ethics. The Code of Ethics contains guidelines for responsibilities to the public and to the profession. These guidelines highlight qualities such as honesty, integrity, and respect of privacy (see figure 1.2).

Looking Towards the Future

The field of personal training is expected to continue to grow in the coming years, at faster rates than the average occupation.[12] With the current health status of the U.S. population in mind, the expectation that chronic diseases and disabilities will continue to rise

---

Figure 1.2: Code of Ethics for the American College of Sports Medicine Certified Professional[14]

Responsibility to the Public
- ACSMCPs shall be dedicated to providing competent and legally permissible services within the scope of the KSAs of their respective credential. These services shall be provided with integrity, competence, diligence, and compassion.
- ACSMCPs provide exercise information in a manner that is consistent with evidence-based science and medicine.
- ACSMCPs respect the rights of clients, colleagues, and healthcare professionals, and shall safeguard client confidences within the boundaries of the law.
- Information relating to the ACSMCP-client relationship is confidential and may not be communicated to a third party not involved in that client's care without the prior written consent of the client or as required by law.
- ACSMCPs are truthful about their qualifications and the limitations of their expertise and provide services consistent with their competencies.

Responsibility to the Profession
- ACSMCPs maintain high professional standards. As such, an ACSMCP should never represent himself or herself, either directly or indirectly, as anything other than an ACSMCP unless he or she holds other license/certification that allows him or her to do so.
- ACSMCPs practice within the scope of their KSAs. ACSMCPs will not provide services that are limited by state law to provision by another healthcare professional only.
- An ACSMCP must remain in good standing relative to governmental requirements as a condition of continued credentialing.
- ACSMCPs take credit, including authorship, only for work they have actually performed and give credit to the contributions of others as warranted.
- Consistent with the requirements of their certification or registration, ACSMCPs must complete approved, additional educational course work aimed at maintain and advancing their KSAs.

---

in the coming years, and the understanding that there are different considerations that must be made for different populations, additional training in "specialty" areas has become more important. Recognizing this, ACSM has partnered with other organizations to launch a series of "Specialty Certifications" that include the ACSM/ACS Certified Cancer Exercise Trainer (CET), ACSM/NCHPAD Certified Inclusive Fitness Trainer (CIFT), and ACSM/NSPAPPH Physical Activity in Public Health Specialist (PAPHS).[11] These additional certifications both (1) broaden the personal trainer's client-base and (2) prepare the individual to have an impact in populations that are growing in size but remain under-served.

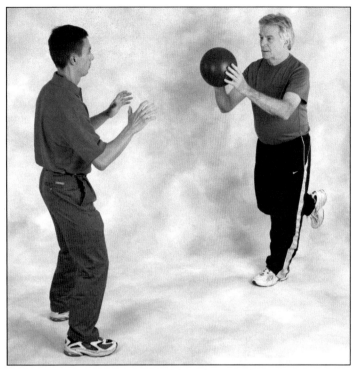

© 2010 American College of Sports Medicine. Used with permission.

References

1. Wu SY, Green A. Projection of chronic illness prevalence and cost inflation. Santa Monica, CA: RAND Health; 2000.

2. National Center for Chronic Disease Prevention and Health Promotion. (2010). Chronic disease prevention and health promotion. *Centers for Disease Control and Prevention.* September 24, 2011. From http://www.cdc.gov/chronicdisease/overview/index.htm.

3. Kung HC, Hoyert DL, Xu JQ, Murphy SL. Deaths: final data for 2005. National Vital Statistics Reports 2008;56(10). Available from: http://www.cdc.gov/nchs/data/nvsr/nvsr56/nvsr56_10.pdf

4. U.S. Department of Health and Human Services. Office of Disease Prevention and Health Promotion. *Healthy People 2020.* Washington, DC. Available at http://www.healthypeople.gov/2020/default.aspx. Accessed September 24, 2011.

5. U.S. Department of Health and Human Services. (2008). 2008 physical activity guidelines for Americans summary. *Physical Activity Guidelines for Americans.* September 24, 2011. From http://www.health.gov/PAGuidelines/guidelines/summary.aspx .

6 Rimmer, J., Riley, B., Wang, E., Rauworth, A. & Jurkowski, J. (2004). Physical activity participation among persons with disabilities: Barriers and facilitators. *American Journal of Preventive Medicine,* 26(5), 419-425.

7. McClaran, S. (2003). The effectiveness of personal training on changing attitudes towards physical activity. *Journal of Sports Science and Medicine,* 2, 10-14.

8. Jeffery, R., Wing, R., Thorson, C. & Burton, L. (1998). Use of personal trainers and financial incentives to increase exercise in a behavioral weight loss program. *Journal of Consulting and Clinical Psychology,* 66(5), 777-783.

9. Mazzetti, S., Kraemer, W., Volek, J., Duncan, N., Ratamess, N., Gomez, A., Newton, R., Hakkinen, K. & Fleck, S. (2000). The influence of direct supervision of resistance training on strength performance. *Medicine and Science in Sports and Exercise,* 32(6), 1175-1184.

10. Maloof, R., Zabik, R. & Dawson, M. (2001). The effect of use of a personal trainer on improvement of health-related fitness in adults (Abstract only). *Medicine and Science in Sports and Exercise,* 33(5) Supplement 1, s74.

11. American College of Sports Medicine. (2007). Certification and Workshops. *American College of Sports Medicine.* September 24, 2011. From http://www.acsm.org/AM/Template.cfm?Section=Certification_Home&Template=/CM/HTMLDisplay.cfm&ContentID=15804

12. United States Department of Labor. (2009). Occupational outlook handbooks, 2010-11 edition: Fitness workers. *Bureau of Labor Statistics.* September 24, 2011. From http://www.bls.gov/oco/ocos296.htm.

13. Institute for Credentialing Excellence. (2009). National Commission on Certifying Agencies. Retrieved from http://www.credentialingexcellence.org/ProgramsandEvents/NCCAAccreditation/tabid/82/Default.aspx.

14. American College of Sports Medicine. (2009). ACSM's Resources for the Personal Trainer: 3rd edition. Lippincott, Williams & Wilson.

15. United States Department of Labor. (2011). Occupational employment statistics: Occupational employment and wages, May 2010. *Bureau of Labor Statistics.* September 24, 2011. From http://www.bls.gov/oes/current/oes399031.htm.

16. American Council on Exercise. (2011). 2010 Salary Survey Results. *American Council on Exercise.* September 24, 2011. From http://www.acefitness.org/salary/.

CHAPTER 2

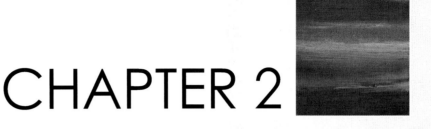

Need for Certified Inclusive Fitness Trainers

By Jennifer N. Green, M.S.

Jennifer Green, M.S., holds a Bachelors of Science degree from Central Michigan University where she majored in Health Fitness in Preventative and Rehabilitative Programs and a Masters of Science degree from Benedictine University in Clinical Exercise Physiology. Upon completion of her masters degree Jennifer worked for the National Center on Physical Activity (www.nchpad.org) and Disability in the Department of Disability and Human Development at the University of Illinois at Chicago.

Jennifer has been heavily involved in the training and educational workshops held for the Certified Inclusive Fitness Trainer certification offered through the American College of Sports Medicine. In addition, Jennifer serves as the staff liaison for the Inclusive Fitness Coalition (www.incfit.org).

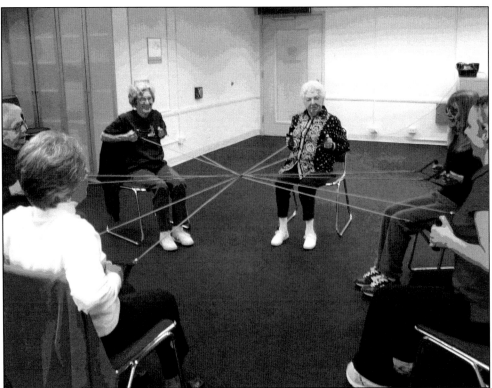

Why Inclusive Fitness Trainers?

People with disabilities (PWD) are one of the largest subgroups in the United States with over 50 million people (approximately 20%) reporting some type of disability.[2] This figure is continuously increasing through population growth, medical advances and the aging process.[3] Disability goes beyond just those with a diagnosed condition; it can also include groups such as aging Baby Boomers as well as anyone with an activity limitation. A large number of health disparities tend to occur within this populace. Thus, a greater number of effective strategies are needed to improve, as well as maintain, daily function and quality of life such as enhanced access and participation in community fitness settings. Despite the enormous health benefits that can be attained from regular physical activity, most individuals with disabilities are not achieving the U.S. recommended goal of 30 minutes a day of moderate intensity physical activity, five or more days of the week.[1,5-7,10,11] Such low levels of physical activity involvement are an even larger concern for PWD when compared to a fairly sedentary population devoid of existing comorbidities. Individuals with disabilities frequently deal with other health issues related to their disability such as secondary conditions (*e.g.,* obesity, pressure sores, hypertension, pain, deconditioning) and associated conditions (*e.g.,* spasticity, autonomic dysfunction, seizures, thermoregulatory issues).[4,6] When these conditions overlay chronic conditions such as type 2 diabetes or heart disease, health becomes an exceptionally significant concern for millions of people with disabilities and their capacity to live independently as well as maintain their connection to society.[8] As a result, increasing physical activity involvement among PWD is an important goal for the health and fitness profession.

Barriers to Physical Activity

While regular physical activity has the potential to offset some of the decline in health and function observed in people with disabilities, barriers to promoting increased participation must first be addressed.[10] Barriers that have often been reported by people with disabilities include cost of fitness center memberships, lack of transportation, lack of information on available and accessible facilities and programs, lack of accessible exercise equipment that can be purchased for home use, and the perception that fitness facilities are unfriendly environments for those who stray from the visual "norm" of what many consider a typical fitness facility patron. Barriers such as these can result in insufficient levels of physical activity participation and a decline in physical function.[5, 7] There is a strong call to action for health and fitness professionals to address these barriers and have the knowledge to create safe and effective exercise programs for people with disabilities. Certified Inclusive Fitness Trainers (CIFTs) have a unique opportunity to impact a substantial sector of the population who are underutilizing facilities designed for fitness and recreation as well as recreation opportunities within their communities.

The Certified Inclusive Fitness Trainer

The CIFT has the knowledge to systematically address physical activity barriers experienced by individuals with disabilities through increased access, participation and adherence. The Certified Inclusive Fitness Trainer understands that access is necessary for participation, and regular participation and adherence are necessary to obtain benefits in health and function.[9] Numerous individuals benefit from this specialty certification. Fitness facilities are able to reach a larger, more diverse clientele by addressing physical, programmatic and attitudinal barriers when a CIFT is available. Individuals with disabilities are able to achieve higher levels of physical activity and substantial health benefits when more opportunities for fitness and active leisure participation are presented to them.

Professionals working in the health and fitness industry must recognize the low rates of physical activity reported among PWD and begin to develop effective and cohesive strategies that address this issue. While these strategies must include proper training in order to create safe environments; the continued growth of inclusive fitness is dependent upon CIFTs and their knowledge of the broader advocacy and policy issues as well.

The first step is ensuring fitness professionals are properly trained and educated to work with this population. The body's response to exercise varies greatly when various conditions are present. Professionals must fully understand that these varying responses require particular exercise considerations in order to create and oversee safe and effective programming.

By studying and sitting for the ACSM/NCHPAD Certified Inclusive Fitness Trainer certification, professionals are able to gain knowledge that will allow them to:

(1) understand the prevalence of disability;

(2) understand the need to address disability issues in the field of health, exercise, and fitness;

(3) know the Americans with Disabilities Act (ADA) and how it directly applies to the field;

(4) develop the skills necessary to address disability concerns;

(5) develop an awareness of how disability subgroups differ from one another and from the general public; and

(6) become aware of useful assistive technologies and how to access them.

In all, the opportunities are vast for a fitness professional looking to expand their level of expertise. The continued growth of inclusive fitness is truly dependent on Certified Inclusive Fitness Trainers and their understanding of the broader issues, not just exercise prescription knowledge. With the help of a CIFT, many of the issues that are often associated with sedentary lifestyles for PWD can be addressed and independence can be maintained.

References

1. CDC. Physical activity among adults with a disability-United States, 2005. MMWR 2007;56:1021-1024.

2. Centers for Disease Control and Prevention. Prevalence of disabilities and associated health conditions among adults–United States, 1999. MMWR Morb Mortal Wkly Rep. 50, 120-125, 2001.

3. Disability and Health. (2011). Retrieved September 23, 2011, from http://www.who.int/mediacentre/factsheets/fs352/en/index.html

4. Rimmer, JH. (2008). Promoting inclusive physical activity communities for people with disabilities Series 9, No. 2. Washington, D.C.: President's Council on Physical Fitness and Sports Washington, D.C.

5. Rimmer JH. The conspicuous absence of people with disabilities in public fitness and recreation facilities: lack of interest or lack of access? Am J Health Promot 2005; 19:327-329.

6. Rimmer JH. Use of the ICF in identifying factors that impact participation in physical activity/rehabilitation among people with disabilities. Dis & Rehabil 2006; 28(17):1087-1095

7. Rimmer JH, Riley B, Wang E, Rauworth A, Jurkowski J. Physical Activity participation among persons with disabilities: barriers and facilitators. Am J Prev Med 2004; 26(5):419-425

8. Rimmer JH, Rowland JL. Health Promotion for people with disabilities: Implications for empowering the person and promoting disability-friendly environments. Am J Lifestyle Med, 2008; 2(5):409-420

9. Rimmer JH, Schiller WJ. Future directions in exercise and recreational technology for people with spinal cord injury and other disabilities: Perspectives from the Rehabilitation Engineering Research Center on Disabilities. Top Spinal Cord Injury Rehabil 2006; 11:82-93

10. Rimmer JH, Shenoy SS. Impact of exercise on targeted secondary conditions. In: Field MJ, Jette AM, Martin L, editors. Workshop on disability in America. Washington DC: National Academies Press; 2006.

11. Wilber N, Mitra M, Walker D, et al. Disability as a public health issue: findings and reflections from the Massachusetts survey of secondary conditions. Milbank Q 2002; 80:393-421.

CHAPTER 3

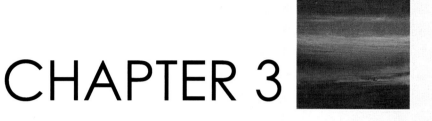

Career Paths for the Certified Inclusive Fitness Trainer

By Samantha Blythe Hiss, M.S., RCEP

Blythe Hiss, M.S., RCEP, holds a Bachelor of Science Degree in Biological Sciences (concentration in Nutrition) from North Carolina State University in Raleigh, North Carolina, and a Master of Science degree in Movement Sciences (concentration in Applied Exercise Physiology) from the University of Illinois at Chicago. She received her Registered Clinical Exercise Physiologist certification from the American College of Sports Medicine (ACSM) in May of 2008. Blythe has worked for both the National Center on Health, Physical Activity and Disability (NCHPAD) and the Rehabilitation Engineering Research Center on Exercise Physiology and Recreational Technology for People with Disabilities in the Department of Disability and Human Development at the UIC.

By being eligible to pursue the Certified Inclusive Fitness Trainer (CIFT) specialty certification, you have already met requirements acknowledging that you have a solid foundation in health and fitness competencies. Now the CIFT will address the knowledge, skills, and abilities specifically for applying that competency toward working with individuals who may have a physical, sensory, or cognitive disability. The CIFT is intended for you to support clients at a level consistent with your pre-requisite certification. You are required to stay within the scope of practice consistent with your respective certification as well as the CIFT, if earned, and your clients must be either apparently healthy or cleared by their physician to participate in independent physical activity. But remember, an important component of the CIFT goes beyond physiology. Becoming a CIFT will allow you to develop a greater understanding of disability in general (*i.e.,* someone can have a disability *and* be healthy), providing you with a unique awareness that will be instrumental in empowering and benefiting your clients.

Where Does a Certified Inclusive Fitness Trainer Find Employment?

Work settings for a CIFT may include both mainstream and non-mainstream fitness arenas. The certification may give you an advantage or a desire to find a position in an environment that may have an increased understanding of individuals with disabilities, including individuals with chronic illness, those who are morbidly obese, as well as aging populations where individuals are likely to encounter various activity limitations. Some examples are:

- Medical fitness centers. Medical fitness centers are medically integrated health and fitness facilities growing in number in the U.S. with more than 950 existing currently (http://medicalfitness.org). The Medical Fitness Association (MFA) currently partners with HPCareer.net for the MFA Career Services at http://mfa.hpcareer.net/ in order to provide both individuals and employers a forum for finding career opportunities.

- Residential care facilities. These are environments such as assisted living facilities, retirement communities, personal care facilities, or group homes where they frequently maintain health and wellness programs with onsite exercises facilities.

- Independent living centers. Independent living centers are often non-residential, private, non-profit, consumer-controlled, community-based organizations providing services, including health and wellness programming, and advocacy by and for persons with all types of disabilities (http://www.ilusa.com/links/ilcenters.htm).

- The National Center on Health, Physical Activity and Disability (NCHPAD) lists employment and positions related to physical activity and disability at http://www.nchpad.org as well as offers the opportunity to list your profile in its searchable Personal Trainer Directory.

- The Inclusive Fitness Coalition maintains a listserv that allows you to submit and receive information for potential job postings, as well as to receive announcements regarding coalition activities and inclusive fitness. Visit http://lists.incfit.org/mailman/listinfo/incfit_listserv for more information.

The CIFT will also set you apart in more mainstream fitness venues where less specialized trainers may not have the knowledge and skills to comfortably and safely work with individuals who have a physical, sensory, or cognitive disability. These more mainstream settings may include community and public health settings such as YMCAs, parks & recreation departments, and after-school programs, commercial health clubs, corporate wellness centers, university recreation centers, or even country clubs and resorts. Having a CIFT provide services at a mainstream fitness facility can help minimize the number and types of barriers that people with disabilities have reported in these environments including environmental, attitudinal, and programmatic barriers.[1]

A CIFT can hold various positions within these work settings, positions that are not unlike those of non-CIFT certified trainers, but the knowledge, skills, and abilities of a CIFT can provide a platform for more responsibility, advancement, or bargaining power for higher pay. Your new skills can help your facility attract and retain clients by providing an onsite contact that understands the importance of, and methods for, creating a more inviting and inclusive environment for everyone. Facilities may create their own unique title or position for those who have this training and can use their expertise to ensure facility policies, procedures, programs, and environments are safe, effective, and conducive to attracting and retaining a wide variety of clientele. Some career resources in more mainstream settings include:

- American College of Sports Medicine® (ACSM)
  ✔ http://www.acsm.org/find-continuing-education/career-resources

- If you hold an ACSM certification, you may also list your profile on its searchable "ProFinder" directory at:
  ✔ http://members.acsm.org/source/custom/Online_locator/onlineLocatorSignup.cfm

- The American Council on Exercise® (ACE)
  ✔ http://www.GymJOB.com

- If you hold an ACE certification, you may also list your profile on their searchable directory at:
  ✔ http://www.acefitness.org/findanacepro/default.aspx

- The National Academy of Sports Medicine® (NASM)
  ✔ http://www.nasmfitjobs.com/a/jobs/find-jobs

- YMCA
  ✔ http://www.ymca.net/career-opportunities/

- JCC (Jewish Community Center)
  ✔ http://www.jccworks.com/

- IHRSA (the International Health, Racquet & Sportsclub Association)
  ✔ http://www.ihrsa.org/careers/Re

The Fitness Job Market

Even though the U.S. job market has declined, employment for fitness professionals is expected to grow much faster than the average (29%) and job prospects are expected to be good through 2018.[2] This is due to: (1) continued job growth in health clubs, fitness facilities, and other similar settings, (2) the increasing number of people who are spending time and money on fitness, and (3) more businesses who are recognizing the benefits of health and fitness programs for their employees. Aging baby boomers (with accompanying aging "ailments" that fitness professionals will need to address) will contribute largely to this employment growth as retiring baby boomers are expected to have more leisure time, higher disposable incomes, and more concern for health and fitness than previous generations.[2] Though this growth is good news, we should expect to face tough competition for jobs and those with formal and/or specialized training will have the best chances. You need to set yourself apart, and that's what the CIFT does.

As more and more people, both with and without disabilities, recognize that healthy eating and regular exercise are vital to a longer, healthier life, job opportunities for fitness professionals that are willing and knowledgeable to assist them will continue to grow. The "I" in CIFT is for "inclusive," which simply put, means including everyone. Fitness professionals can, and should, learn ways to be inclusive in their facilities and in their testing and programming methods. The demand for inclusive fitness has grown tremendously over the past few years however it is only with continued advocacy on behalf of the fitness professionals that fitness facilities and equipment manufacturers will invest more resources to make equipment, programming, services, and job opportunities readily available and appropriate to meet the needs of people with disabilities.

References:

1. Rimmer, J., Riley, B., Wang, E., Rauworth, A. & Jurkowski, J. (2004). Physical activity participation among persons with disabilities: Barriers and facilitators. American Journal of Preventive Medicine, 26(5), 419-425.

2. United States Department of Labor. (2009). Occupational outlook handbooks, 2010-11 edition: Fitness workers. Bureau of Labor Statistics. September 26, 2011. From http://www.bls.gov/oco/ocos296.htm.

Section II

Americans with Disabilities Act (ADA): Applications, Policies, and Principals

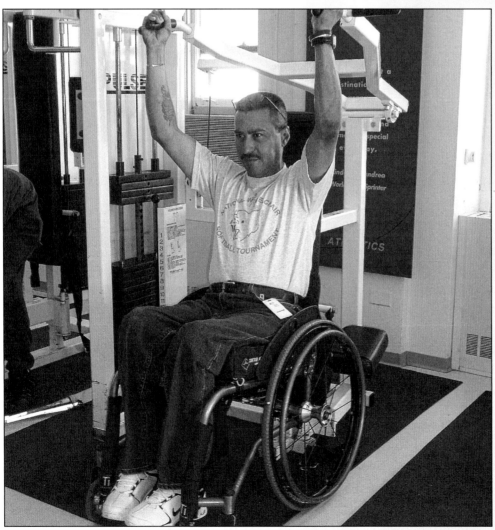

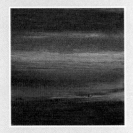

CHAPTER 4

ADA Background and History:

The Americans With Disabilities Act of 1990, Public Law 101-336

By Chris Mackey, B.S., CFT

Chris Mackey has a bachelor's degree in Therapeutic Recreation from East Carolina University and is an ISSA Certified Fitness Trainer. He was born with Spina Bifida and has participated in wheelchair sports, including competitive swimming and wheelchair basketball. He also has worked as the Healthy Communities Coordinator for the North Carolina Office on Disability and Health at the University of North Carolina at Chapel Hill, Chapel Hill, NC. He has more than a decade of experience working in accessible community design, Americans with Disabilities Act requirements and Universal Design principles.

The Americans with Disabilities Act (ADA) is a landmark piece of civil rights legislation that provides sweeping protections and a basic level of access for people with disabilities in the United States. Signed into law by President George H. W. Bush on July 26, 1990, the ADA was a significant accomplishment of the Disability Rights Movement, which was modeled after the Civil Rights Movement. The passage of the ADA involved decades of activism and advocacy on the part of people with disabilities and their supporters who demanded desegregation of people with disabilities and equal access to employment, public transportation, and the removal of architectural and programmatic barriers that prevent participation in community life.[1]

The ADA was preceded by, and in many ways modeled after, several pieces of legislation that gradually gave people with disabilities in the U.S. rights to various federal programs. These laws date back as far as the late 1960s, beginning with the passage of the Architectural Barriers Act of 1968 (ABA) P.L. 90-480, which requires all buildings of the federal government to be accessible to people with disabilities. The ABA set standards for building accessibility that are very similar to the ones developed for the ADA. Several other pieces of legislation followed the passage of the ABA. Section 504 of the Rehabilitation Act of 1973 banned discrimination on the basis of disability in all federally funded programs, including public schools. Public Law 94-142, the Education for All Handicapped Children Act was passed in 1975 and became the Individuals with Disabilities Education Act (IDEA), a U.S. Federal Law establishing what is commonly known as Special Education. This law, like Section 504, afforded students with disabilities a "free and appropriate public education." Other laws included the Air Carrier Access Act of 1986 (49 U.S.C. § 41705) and the Fair Housing Act as amended in 1988, (42 U.S.C. §§ 3601) that prohibits discrimination on the basis of disability in the provision of air travel and housing. The recreation portions of the reauthorization of the Rehabilitation act in 2003 and the Improved Nutrition and Physical Activity Act were also designed to provide more opportunities to prevent obesity for children and adults. Before and since the passage of the ADA, other disability rights laws have been passed to address inequities in other aspects of the lives of people with disabilities.[2]

References

1. Mayerson, Arlene. The Americans With Disabilities Act of 1990: A Movement Perspective. Disability Rights Education Defense Fund, (DREDF), 1992. Downloaded September 2011 from http://dredf.org/publications/ada_history.shtml

2. United States Department of Justice Civil Rights Division, Disability Rights Section (2005). A Guide to Disability Rights Laws . . Downloaded at http://www.ada.gov/cguide.pdf.

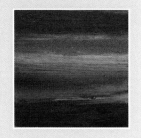

CHAPTER 5

Promoting Basic Accessibility:

The ADA and Fitness Facilities

By Chris Mackey, B.S., CFT

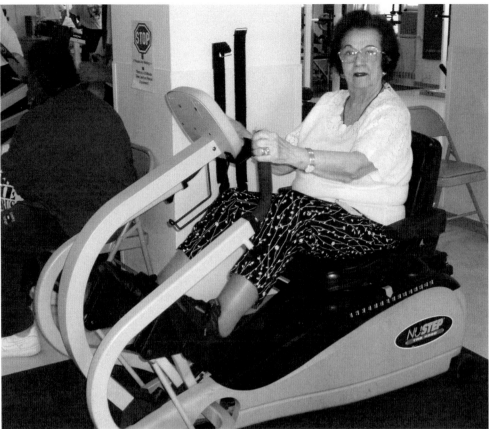

Who is Protected by the ADA?

The ADA as written referrs to a three-prong definition of disability.[1] If an individual falls under one of the following categories, he or she has rights under and is protected by the ADA: (1) A person who has a physical or mental impairment that substantially limits one or more major life activity, such as speaking, walking, caring for oneself, hearing, learning, or concentrating. Included in this definition are also people who have limitations in one or more major bodily function, such as respiratory, endocrine, immune or reproductive functions. (2) A person who has a record of such impairment, such as someone who has a history of cancer or Multiple Sclerosis. (3) A person who is regarded as having such an impairment. If someone is discriminated against because of a feature or condition that is not substantially limiting a major life activity, they are protected under this prong of the definition. For example, a person who has a facial disfigurement who is denied participation in a program may not be substantially limited in a life activity, but has a physical attribute that caused discrimination to take place.[2]

The Titles of the ADA

The ADA expanded on, and perhaps filled in the gaps left by previous disability rights laws, which dealt mainly with programs and services offered by the federal government.

It is comprised of five parts, or Titles, each of which prohibits discrimination on the basis of disability in a particular area not covered.

Title I: Employment

Title I of the ADA states that employers with 15 or more employees can not discriminate on the basis of disability in their hiring and firing practices. Employers must also make reasonable accommodations for employees with disabilities so they are able to do their jobs. This could mean providing a flexible work schedule or providing certain assistive technologies, as long as doing so does not pose undue hardship on the employer/organization. Title I also restricts the types of questions a potential employer may ask regarding disability during an interview process. It is important to note here that Title I not only protects an individual with a disability seeking employment, but also an individual seeking employment who is affiliated with a person who has a disability. This means that if a parent of a child with a disability needs accommodations, such as a flexible work schedule or time off to take care of their child, they are covered by or have rights under Title I.

Title II State or Local Government Entities

Title II of the ADA requires that people with disabilities be given equal opportunity to take part in state or local government programs (e.g., state or local parks and recreation programs, state universities, or local health department programs). State or local government entities must make reasonable modifications to policies, practices and procedures so that people with disabilities can participate, unless they can show that doing so would (1) Fundamentally alter the service provided, (e.g., change the nature of an activity); (2) Pose a danger to others; or (3) Pose an undue administrative or financial burden on the agency, (e.g., not enough money or one-to-one staffing where it might be needed). At a minimum, state and local government programs must also follow the ADA Standards for Accessible Design (which will be discussed later) when building new or renovating older buildings. Title II entities must also provide effective communication to participants with communication disabilities, which can include the provision of sign language interpreters for participants who are deaf.

Title II Transportation Provisions:

Title II also prohibits discrimination on the basis of disability by public transportation organizations. This includes modifications of policies, practices and procedures, provision of accessible vehicles and paratransit or transit that is provided for those who cannot access mainline services.

Title III: Public Accommodations

Title III covers private entities operating places of public accommodation or commercial facilities. It governs access to almost any kind of business, including restaurants, movie theaters, stores, stadiums and privately owned fitness gyms. It also covers transportation services provided by public accommodations and courses and examinations related to professional, educational, or trade-related applications, licensing, certifications, or credentialing. Private health clubs, or gyms, and other Title III entities must make reasonable modifications to their policies, practices and procedures to ensure access for patrons with disabilities. They must also at a minimum follow the ADA Standards for Accessible Design in designing new or renovating old facilities and remove any barriers to participation by patrons with disabilities as long as doing so can be done without too much difficulty or expense. This is also known as Readily Achievable Barrier Removal. What is readily achievable is determined on a case-by-case basis, depending on the covered entity's (mainly) financial resources and current building conditions. Examples of readily achievable barrier removal could be moving equipment, putting in a curb cut, lowering door pressures, or lowering dispensers in restrooms. As with Title II entities, Title III entities are not required to remove barriers if doing so would pose a danger to others or fundamentally alter the services provided. For example, a facility would not have to pave a beach volleyball court as that would be a fundamental alteration of the sport of beach volleyball.[3]

Title IV: Telecommunications

Title IV of the ADA established the interstate telecommunications relay system. This allows for individuals with communication disabilities to use a teletypewriter (TTY) to communicate with someone who is using a regular phone through a trained operator.

Title V: Miscellaneous Provisions

Title V of the ADA covers areas not covered in the other four titles or other laws. For example, it governs access to wilderness areas and facilities of Congress. It also prohibits coercion or retaliation related to ADA complaints. For example, a health club or fitness center cannot coerce a member with a disability into not filing an ADA complaint (coercion) or revoke a patron's membership for filing an ADA complaint (retaliation).

The 2010 ADA Standards for Accessible Design

As of March 15, 2012, entities covered under the ADA must incorporate what are known as the 2010 ADA Standards for Accessible Design into their newly designed, existing, or altered facilities. The ADA is unique in that it is a civil rights law that mainly focuses on architectural barriers, and the ADA Standards for Accessible Design are the requirements that specify how (primarily) the built environment of any covered entity must be designed so that it is accessible. Some of the requirements of the ADA Standards[4] include:

- At least one 60 inch diameter circle to allow for turning around by patrons in wheelchair or scooter
- A 30 inch x 48 inch area of clear floor space next to a piece of equipment

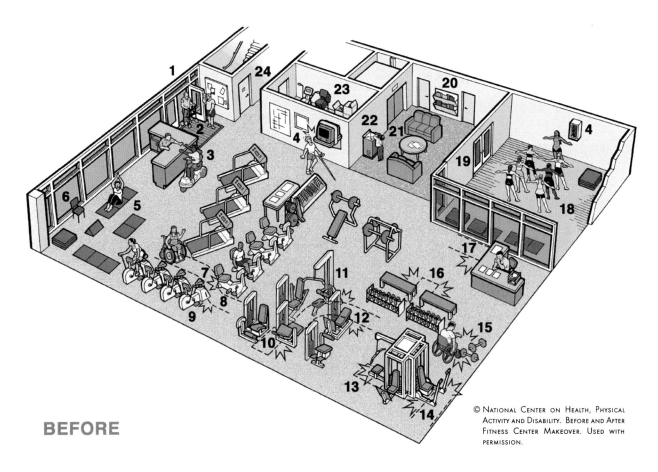

BEFORE

© National Center on Health, Physical Activity and Disability. Before and After Fitness Center Makeover. Used with permission.

so patrons have room for assistive devices. This space should be positioned next to the seat or appropriate transfer point.

- Locker rooms with accessible shower stalls (3 feet x 3 feet) and wheelchair-accessible toilet stalls (5 feet x 5 feet)
- Reception and other counter space no higher than 36 inches
- Providing sign language interpreter services at no charge (provided enough advance notice is given)
- Allowing a personal attendant at no charge into the facility to assist with changing clothes and other personal care
- Doors that require less that 5 pounds of force to open
- A pool with an accessible entrance such as a lift or pool stairs
- Placing at least one of every piece of equipment along an accessible route
- Placing equipment at the end of a row for easier access

Information on ADA and Enforcement

The U.S. Department of Justice, (USDOJ), is the lead enforcement agency for the Americans with Disabilities Act and the 2010 ADA Standards for Accessible Design. In some cases other federal agencies enforce ADA provisions that apply to areas they govern, such as the Equal Employment Opportunities Commission enforces the Title I/employment provisions of the ADA. For information regarding a facility's obligations under the ADA,

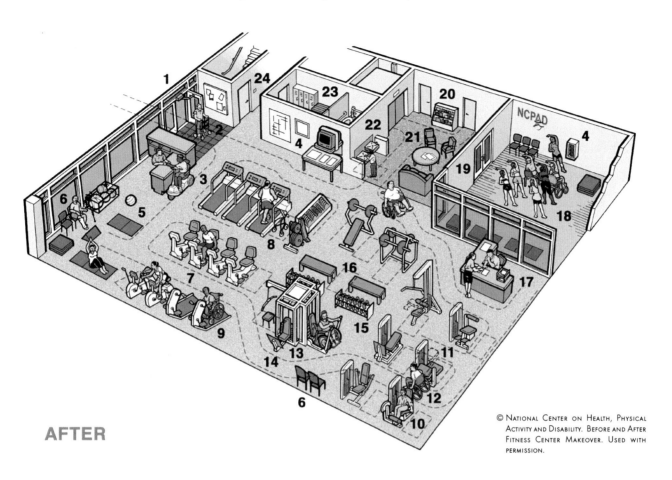

AFTER

© National Center on Health, Physical Activity and Disability. Before and After Fitness Center Makeover. Used with permission.

the USDOJ has a web site, www.ada.gov, and a hotline 1(800) 514-0301 or 1(800) 514-0383 (TTY). Another resource for information on accessible design is the U.S. Architectural and Transportation Barriers Compliance Board, also known as the U.S. Access Board, www.access-board.gov. The Access Board is the agency which develops what is known as the ADA Accessibility Guidelines, or ADAAG. This development process can last for several years and involves input from builders and designers, members of the business community, people with disabilities and disability advocates. Once a final set of ADA Accessibility Guidelines is created, it is sent to the USDOJ for further review and then signed into law. So what eventually becomes the ADA Standards for Accessible Design starts its development at the Access Board. Both the Access Board and the USDOJ ADA Web site (www.ada.gov) can provide guidance to a fitness center's staff on questions about improving access for persons with disabilities.

References

1. United States Department of Justice Civil Rights Division, Disability Rights Section (2005). A Guide to Disability Rights Laws . . Downloaded at http://www.ada.gov/cguide.pdf.

2. Southwest ADA Center. Disability Law Handbook. Downloaded at:http://www.dlrp.org/html/publications/dlh/overview.html

3. McGovern, John N., JD. Recreation Access Rights Under the ADA. Downloaded from the National Center on Accessibility at http://www.indiana.edu/~nca/nchpad/rights.shtml .

4. North Carolina Office on Disability and Health (2008). Removing Barriers to Health Clubs and Fitness Facilities. Chapel Hill, NC: FPG Child Development Institute.

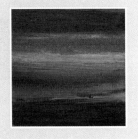

CHAPTER 6

Universal Design in Fitness Facilities

By Chris Mackey, B.S., CFT

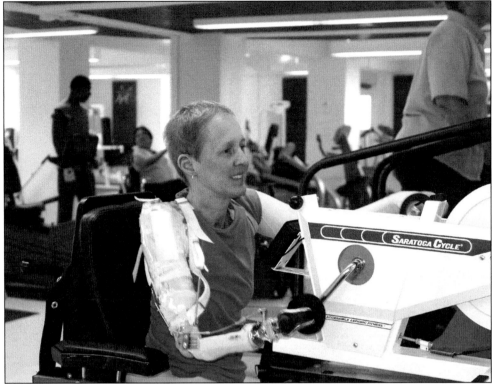

The ADA and other accessibility statutes provide only a minimum level of access to any fitness facility. To ensure that people with disabilities can fully participate in the programs and services of any fitness center, it should incorporate principles of Universal Design. This term, coined by architect Ronald L. Mace, describes environments that go beyond the requirements of accessibility laws and is defined as: **"The design of products and environments to be usable by all people, to the greatest extent possible, without the need for adaptation or specialized design."**[1]

Any space, equipment, or program in a fitness center that incorporates Universal Design should follow seven principles and accompanying guidelines:[1]

Principle 1: Equitable use

The design is useful and marketable to people with diverse abilities, such as:

1a. Providing the same means of use for all users: identical whenever possible; equivalent when not.

1b. Avoiding segregating or stigmatizing any users.

1c. Including provisions for privacy, security, and safety should be equally available to all users.

1d. Making the design appealing to all users.

Principle 2: Flexibility in Use

The design accommodates a wide range of individual preferences and abilities, and:

2a. Provides a choice for methods of use.

2b. Accommodates right- or left-handed access and use.

2c. Facilitates a user's accuracy and precision.

2d. Provides adaptability to the user's pace.

Principle 3: Simple and Intuitive Use

Use of the design is easy to understand, regardless of the user's experience, knowledge, language skills, or current concentration level. It does/is:

3a. Eliminate unnecessary complexity.

3b. Consistent with user expectations and intuition.

3c. Accommodate a wide range of literacy and language skills.

3d. Arrange information consistent with its importance.

3e. Provide effective prompting and feedback during and after task completion.

Principle 4: Perceptible Information

The design communicates necessary information effectively to the user, regardless of ambient conditions or the user's sensory abilities. The design:

4a. Uses different modes (pictorial, verbal, tactile) for redundant presentation of essential information.

4b. Provides adequate contrast between essential information and its surroundings.

4c. Maximizes "legibility" of essential information.

4d. Differentiates elements in ways that can be described (i.e., make it easy to give instructions or directions).

4e. Provides compatibility with a variety of techniques or devices used by people with sensory limitations.

Principle 5: Tolerance for Error

The design minimizes hazards and the adverse consequences of accidental or unintended actions. It:

5a. Arranges elements to minimize hazards and errors: most used elements, most accessible; hazardous elements eliminated, isolated, or shielded.

5b. Provides warnings of hazards and errors.

5c. Provides fail safe features.

5d. Discourages unconscious action in tasks that require vigilance.

Principle 6: Low Physical Effort

The design can be used efficiently and comfortably and with a minimum of fatigue, and:

6a. Allows user to maintain a neutral body position.

6b. Uses reasonable operating forces.

6c. Minimizes repetitive actions.

6d. Minimizes sustained physical effort.

Principle 7: Size and Space for Approach and Use

Appropriate size and space is provided for approach, reach, manipulation, and use regardless of user's body size, posture, or mobility. The design:

7a. Provides a clear line of sight to important elements for any seated or standing user.

7b. Makes reach to all components comfortable for any seated or standing user.

7c. Accommodates variations in hand and grip size.

7d. Provides adequate space for the use of assistive devices or personal assistance.

Having equipment, a built environment, and programming that is designed with these principles in mind ensures that the greatest number of people, with the widest range of abilities, can take part in a fitness center.[1]

How Can Universal Design Be Applied to a Health Club or Fitness Facility?

Examples of how a fitness facility can incorporate principles of universal design include:

- Accessible multi- and single-station strength equipment
- An aquatic wheelchair for transferring patrons into the pool
- Power doors at entrances
- Chairs in exercise classes to allow someone to participate while seated
- Weight machines with small weight increments

Choosing and Placing Accessible Fitness Equipment

The ADA and other accessibility laws do not specify what equipment fitness facilities must have, only how it should be arranged. The law requires that at least one of each type of equipment be placed along an accessible (at least 36 inch wide) route and that a minimum clear floor space of 30 inch x 48 inch be next to each piece of equipment to allow for room for an assistive device and transferring. Put another way, every unique piece of equipment should be placed along an accessible route. For example, there may be both dumbbells and a Preacher Curl/Bicep Curl machine in a facility. Even though they both exercise the same muscle groups, patrons with disabilities have the right to access all of the equipment options in a facility. When it comes to choosing accessible equipment, fitness facilities should consider those pieces that incorporate Universal Design and select a wide variety of equipment to accommodate diverse abilities.

Many elements go into making exercise equipment in a facility accessible to patrons with disabilities. Consider the following for strength training options and review the accompanying fitness floor diagrams. Figure 1 incorporates both elements of Universal Design and ADA requirements previously mentioned.

Figure 1. Both elements of Universal Design and ADA requirements

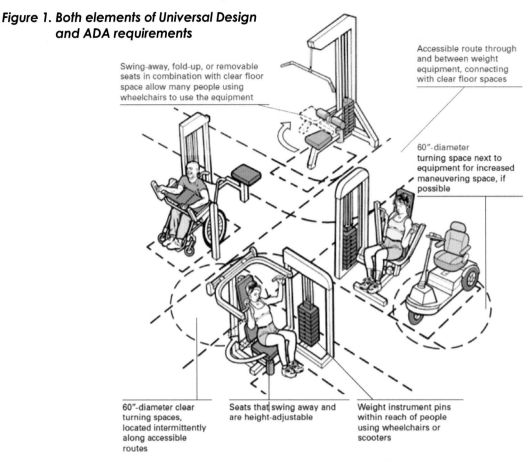

Swing-away, fold-up, or removable seats in combination with clear floor space allow many people using wheelchairs to use the equipment

Accessible route through and between weight equipment, connecting with clear floor spaces

60"-diameter turning space next to equipment for increased maneuvering space, if possible

60"-diameter clear turning spaces, located intermittently along accessible routes

Seats that swing away and are height-adjustable

Weight instrument pins within reach of people using wheelchairs or scooters

- A variety of free weights, including cuff weights for patrons with limited grips, tubing, and dumbbells
- Weight machines that have lower resistance levels, (1 pound and 2 pound options)
- Machines that provide pneumatic or electromagnetic resistance are easier to use for many people who have diminished fine motor control
- Multi-station strength equipment with a removable seat for use by those in wheelchairs
- Raised mats offer an easy-transfer surface for stretching

Figure 2 shows the elements that make cardio equipment accessible include:
- Different types of exercise bikes and recumbent bikes
- Equipment for both arm and leg exercise
- Treadmills that start at a low MPH setting
- Upper arm ergometer that provides strength training and cardiovascular exercise, (these are available in different configurations)

:

Figure 2. Both elements of Universal Design and ADA requirements

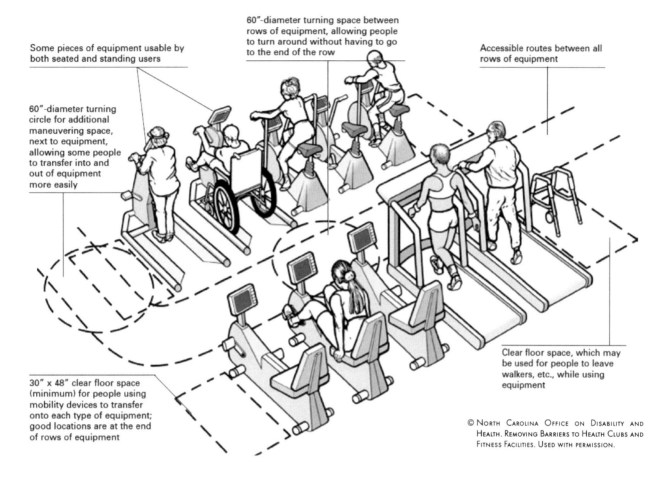

60"-diameter turning space between rows of equipment, allowing people to turn around without having to go to the end of the row

Some pieces of equipment usable by both seated and standing users

Accessible routes between all rows of equipment

60"-diameter turning circle for additional maneuvering space, next to equipment, allowing some people to transfer into and out of equipment more easily

Clear floor space, which may be used for people to leave walkers, etc., while using equipment

30" x 48" clear floor space (minimum) for people using mobility devices to transfer onto each type of equipment; good locations are at the end of rows of equipment

© North Carolina Office on Disability and Health. Removing Barriers to Health Clubs and Fitness Facilities. Used with permission.

Marketing to People with Disabilities:

Remember that the ADA requires that a facility provide effective communication to customers with disabilities. That could mean providing sign language interpreters, alternate formats such as large print, or reading information to patrons with vision impairments or cognitive limitations. Facilities should also design inclusive and accessible marketing campaigns. Consider partnering with disability organizations in your community such as a Center for Independent Living, local Special Olympics programs, or adapted sports team. In creating advertising materials, utilize diverse images, have a written policy statement indicating your facility's willingness to make reasonable accommodations for all people and be compliant with the ADA (figure3).

Offer key materials such as brochures explaining membership fees or the exercise classes you offer in alternate formats, such as large print, (16-18 point font or larger) or Braille. In print and web-based materials, do not use shading, overlays or fancy fonts such as: 𝖋𝖎𝖙𝖓𝖊𝖘𝖘 𝖋𝖆𝖈𝖎𝖑𝖎𝖙𝖞 or *fitness facility*. Do not to use bold or italics and keep your fonts consistent throughout a document.[3]

As you look at improving access in your fitness facility, think of it as a process. An accessibility review should be conducted at least annually and in partnership with individuals with disabilities. Several tools are available. The National Center on Health,

Physical Activity and Disability (NCHPAD has developed Accessibility Instruments Measuring Fitness and Recreation Environments (AIMFREE) tools. These checklists provide both fitness professionals and consumers with a means to evaluate how accessible and welcoming a facility is to patrons with disabilities[4] You may also consult *Removing Barriers to Health Clubs and Fitness Facilities: A Guide for Accommodating All Members, Including People with Disabilities and Older Adults* that has an abbreviated accessibility survey tool for fitness professionals.[5]

For some facilities covered under Title III, there are also tax incentives for removing architectural and transportation barriers. Section 44 of the IRS code provides a tax credit for businesses "who remove access barriers from their facilities, provide accessible services, or take other steps to improve accessibility for customers with disabilities." This applies to businesses with 30 or fewer employees or businesses with less than $1 million in revenue. Under Section 190 of the IRS code, covered businesses may also be eligible for a tax deduction of up to $15,000 for expenses related to barrier removal in facilities or vehicles.[6]

Providing access to your programs and services is the first step, and one that should be continually reviewed . It is important for you to be a voice for inclusion in your fitness facility and ensure that all employees you interact with have an understanding of some basic ways to maintain an accessible facility and where they can seek more information.

References:

1. Center for Universal Design, North Carolina State University. Principles of Universal Design. Downloaded at: http://www.ncsu.edu/project/design-projects/udi/center-for-universal-design/the-principles-of-universal-design/ (Version 2.0 © Copyright 1997 NC State University, The Center for Universal Design, an initiative of the College of Design Compiled by advocates of universal design, listed in alphabetical order: Bettye Rose Connell, Mike Jones, Ron Mace, Jim Mueller, Abir Mullick, Elaine Ostroff, Jon Sanford, Ed Steinfeld, Molly Story, & Gregg Vanderheiden

2. North Carolina Office on Disability and Health (2008). Removing Barriers to Health Clubs and Fitness Facilities. Chapel Hill, NC: FPG Child Development Institute.

3. Aries, Arditi, Ph.D. Designing for People with Partial Sight. Lighthouse International. Downloaded at: http://www.lighthouse.org/accessibility/design/accessible-print-design/making-text-legible/

4. National Center on Health, Physical Activity and Disability, (NCHPAD). Accessibility Instruments Measuring Fitness and Recreation Environments.

5. North Carolina Office on Disability and Health (2008). Removing Barriers to Health Clubs and Fitness Facilities. Chapel Hill, NC: FPG Child Development Institute.

6. United States Department of Justice, Civil Rights Division, Disability Rights Section. Expanding Your Market, Tax Incentives for Businesses. Downloaded September 2011 at http://www.ada.gov/taxincent.pdf .

Section III

Health Appraisal: Fitness and Functional Assessment

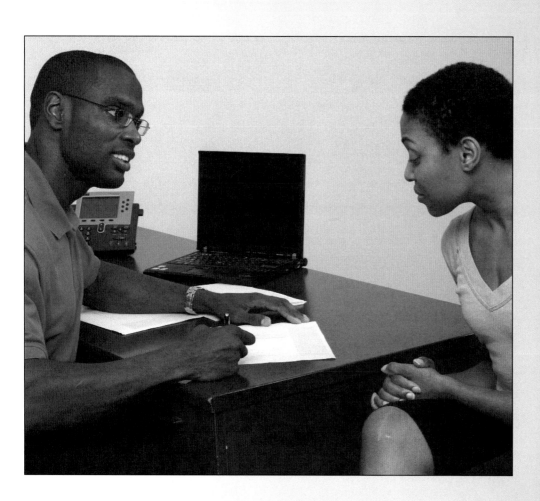

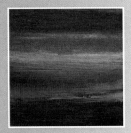

CHAPTER 7

Classification of Function

By Meg Ann Traci, Ph.D.

Meg Ann Traci is a Research Associate Professor at The University of Montana Rural Institute: Center for Excellence in Disabilities Education, Research, and Services.

Increasing Physical Activity Using the International Classification of Functioning, Disability and Health Framework

Individualizing physical activity plans for persons with disabilities is a complex process that may or may not require fitness professionals to develop adaptations or modifications of readily available physical activity options. Hutzler observed this process in physical education settings, and he suggested that "...adaptations cannot be taken as 'off the shelf' solutions, with cookbook type prescriptions of 'if this... then do the following.'"[1] Rather, Hutzler and others (*e.g.,* Andrew, Gabbe, Wolfe, & Cameron, 2010; Hutzler, 2007; Rauworth, 2011; Seekins et al., 2010) recommend using The World Health Organization's (WHO) framework, such as the International Classification of Functioning, Disability and Health (ICF),[2] to support professionals to apply critical thinking to decisions of whether and how to modify physical activities.

The WHO developed the ICF as just one of the systems designed to improve health in the family of 'WHO Family of International Classifications' (http://www.who.int/classifications/en/). Different WHO classifications represent different perspectives on health, and all strive to create a standard common language for describing health from these different perspectives. Fitness professionals may be most familiar with the WHO International Statistical Classification of Diseases and Related Health Problems – 10th Revision (ICD-10) because of its history. The ICD-10 classification creates a standard common language for doctors, epidemiologists, and others who work to prevent or treat disease and other problems (*e.g.,* infections, injuries, conditions), and it describes health from this perspective as the presence or absence of disease and other problems.

The WHO definition of health captures a broader perspective: "Health is a state of complete physical, mental, and social well-being and not merely the absence of disease or infirmity."[3] The ICF (formerly *International Classification of Impairment, Disability and Health*) was developed to describe health as a state of well-being, particularly when and how it exists and does not exist in the presence of disease and other conditions. The ICF is offered as a complement to ICD-10. The demand for the ICF classification has been driven by advances in human service, assistive technology, advocacy, and policy. These advances have given rise to a dramatic increase in the number of people living healthy lives while managing disease or other conditions, including disability.[4] The ICF is "...a classification of health and health-related domains – domains that help us describe changes in body function and structure; what a person with a health condition can do in a standard environment (their level of capacity); as well as what they actually do in their usual environment (their level of performance)."[5] As such, it may be used at individual, institutional, and social planning levels.[5] For fitness professionals, this means the ICF can be used to organize physical activity programs for individuals with disabilities, to improve accessibility and inclusionary aspects of fitness institutions *(e.g.,* fitness centers, sports clubs, parks), and to improve social policy such as standards guiding the development of fitness equipment.

ICF definitions and structure

The ICF classification of health domains and health-related domains is expressed in codes that can create profiles of individuals' functioning, disability and health. "In ICF, the term functioning refers to all body functions, activities and participation, while disability is similarly an umbrella term for impairments, activity limitations and participation restrictions. ICF also lists environmental factors that interact with all these components."[5] An overview of ICF components includes standard definitions for use within the context of health planning:

- *Body functions* are the physiological functions of body systems (including psychological functions).

- *Body structures* are anatomical parts of the body such as organs, limbs, and their components.

- *Impairments* are problems in body function or structure such as a significant deviation or loss.

- *Activity* is the execution of a task or action by an individual.

- *Participation* is involvement in a life situation.[2]

Components of the ICF are grouped into two parts. Part 1, *functioning and disability,* includes body functions and structures as well as activities and participation. Part 2, *contextual factors,* includes environmental factors and personal factors. Figure 1 shows how components of the ICF interact and influence health.

Figure 1. The International Classification of Function.[2]

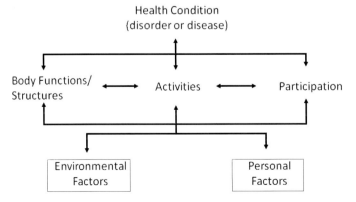

Planning for increased physical activity using the ICF

Programs and interventions designed to increase individuals' physical activity can be described within the ICF framework using a specific code, d5701, for *Managing Diet and Fitness*, from the chapter on Self-Care in the Activities and Participation domain of Part 1 on Functioning and Disability. An individual's *capacity* for (*i.e.,* potential with or without facilitators) and *performance* of (*i.e.,* current status assessed with or without assistive devices) managing diet and fitness activities are qualified using a 5-point scale (0 = "no difficulty"; 2 = "moderate difficulty"; and 4 = "complete difficulty"). Thus someone with current performance difficulties but no anticipated difficulties in their capacity for managing diet and fitness activities could obtain scores of "3" and "0" respectively.

The right side of the ICF model (Figure 1) shows how domains of participation *(e.g.,* remunerative employment; d850) may interact with managing diet and fitness activities. These may be rated for capacity and performance as well. The left side of the ICF model shows how an individual's Body Functions and Structures may interact with managing diet and fitness activities. Hundreds of body functions and structures in eight chapters can be reviewed and relevant ones such as muscle power functions (b730), heart functions (b410), and sleep functions (b134), can be qualified on a 5 point scale (0 = "no impairment"; 2 = "moderate impairment"; and 4 = "complete impairment").

The bottom of the ICF model shows contextual factors interacting with each other and with the interactional processes involving body functions and structures, activities, and participation. Hundreds of ICF contextual factors (*i.e.,* possible facilitators and barriers) are organized into five chapters on (1) products and technology; (2) the natural environment and human-made changes to the environment; (3) support and relationships; (4) attitudes; and (5) services, systems and policies. Importantly, disability and rehabilitation research guided the list of possible contextual factors that may act as facilitators or barriers. As such, the list is somewhat comprehensive, well organized, and described with additional considerations relevant to the experience of disability. Each contextual factor can be qualified as a barrier or as a facilitator using a 5 point scale (0 = "no barrier" or "no facilitator"; 2 = "moderate barrier" or "moderate facilitator"; and 4 = "complete barrier" or "complete facilitator"). In the example of activity qualifiers above, the performance score is less than the capacity score, indicating that some aspect of the environment is a barrier to performance.

Figure 2 is a model developed by Rauworth illustrating how reviews of ICF domains and components can yield recommendations to modify or individualize exercise routines that will be health promoting and sustainable for a stroke survivor.[6] The identification of the effects of the stroke is aided by a review of ICF components in the Body Functions and Structures domain. The existence of barriers is indicated by seemingly lower performance than capacity qualifiers and is confirmed by the identification of environmental and personal factors that are experienced as barriers. Presumably a follow-up assessment using the ICF framework will yield different results and inform a next phase of exercise modifications. Changes in health behavior may improve ability for activities (*e.g.,* using transportation; d470) and ultimately domains of participation (*e.g.,* sports; d9201).

**Figure 2. ICF Model and
Cardiovascular Training
for Stroke Survivors.**[6]

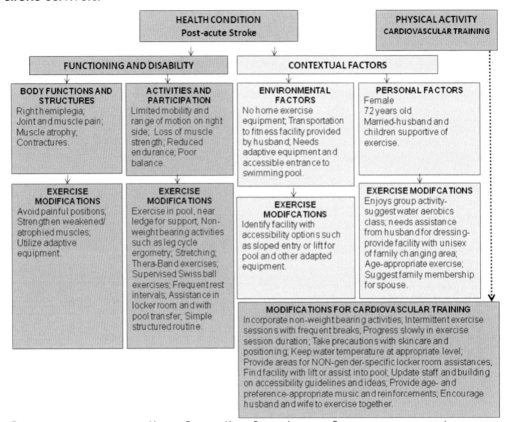

THIS DIAGRAM IS REPRODUCED FROM THE NATIONAL CENTER ON HEALTH, PHYSICAL ACTIVITY AND DISABILITY AT WWW.NCHPAD.ORG. IT MAY BE FREELY DISTRIBUTED IN ITS ENTIRETY AS LONG AS IT INCLUDES THIS NOTICE BUT CANNOT BE EDITED, MODIFIED, OR OTHERWISE ALTERED WITHOUT THE EXPRESS WRITTEN PERMISSION OF NCHPAD. CONTACT NCHPAD AT 1-800-900-8086 FOR ADDITIONAL DETAILS.

Summary

Fitness professionals must consider a myriad of issues when deciding whether and how to modify physical activity options and guidelines for persons with disabilities. The World Health Organization's International Classification of Functioning, Disability and Health can help fitness professionals use a systematic approach to these decisions. The ICF describes health as it exists in the presence or absence of disease and other conditions, taking into consideration function and health with contextual factors in an interactive model. The model is grounded in social-ecological theory that proposes disability as a result of the dynamic interplay of the person and his or her environment. Fitness professionals can review and identify ICF codes to create comprehensive individual profiles for the development of individualized physical activity plans. The ICF also can guide changes to fitness institutions and related social policies to benefit the health and wellness of persons with disabilities.

References

1. Hutzler, Y. A Systematic Ecological Model for Adapting Physical Activities: Theoretical Foundations and Practical Examples. (2007). ADAPTED PHYSICAL ACTIVITY QUARTERLY, 24, 287-304.

2. World Health Organization. (2001). International classification of functioning, disability and health. Geneva: World Health Organization.

3. Preamble to the Constitution of the World Health Organization as adopted by the International Health Conference, New York, 19 June - 22 July 1946; signed on 22 July 1946 by the representatives of 61 States (Official Records of the World Health Organization, no. 2, p. 100) and entered into force on 7 April 1948. The definition has not been amended since 1948.

4. Seelman, K., & Sweeney, S. (1995). The changing universe of disability. American Rehabilitation, Autumn-Winter, 2-13.

5. World Health Organization. (2002). Towards a common language for Functioning, Disability and Health (ICF), Geneva: World Health Organization. Available at: http://www.who.int/classifications/icf/training/icfbeginnersguide.pdf [accessed 31 December, 2011].

6. Rauworth, A. (2006). Use of the International Classification of Functioning, Disability and Health (ICF) to prepare individualized exercise prescriptions for people with disabilities. National Center on Health, Physical Activity and Disabilitynchpad, University of Illinois-Chicago, Chicago, IL. http://www.ncpad.org/fitt/fact_sheet.phpɐsheet=459&view=all

7. Andrew, N. E., Gabbe, B. J., Wolfe, R., and Cameron, P.A. (2010). Evaluation of Instruments for Measuring the Burden of Sport and Active Recreation Injury. Sports Med, 40(2), 141-161.

8. Ravesloot, Rugerio, C. C., Ipsen, C., Traci, M. A., Rigles, B., Boehm, T., Ware, D., and Seekins, T. (2011). Health Behavior Change in the Context of the Disability Experience. Disability and Health Journal, 4, 19-23.

9. Seekins, T., Kimpton, T., Peterson, J., Drum, C. E., Suzuki, R., Heller, T., Krahn, G., McCubbin, J., Rimmer, J., & White, G. (2010). Evidence-Based Health Promotion Interventions for People with Disabilities: Results of a Systematic Review of Literature. Portland, OR: Oregon Health Sciences University, Research and Training Center on Health and Wellness for People with Disabilities.

10. Seelman, K., & Sweeney, S. (1995). The changing universe of disability. American Rehabilitation, Autumn-Winter, 2-13.

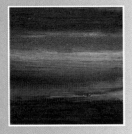

CHAPTER 8

The Initial Client Consultation

By Kirsti Van Dornick, BSc. Kin.;

Bobbi-Jo Atchison, B.P.E.;

and Karen Slater, M.A.

Kirsti Van Dornick is the Athlete Development Coordinator at The Steadward Centre for Personal & Physical Achievement. She holds certifications including CSEP-CEP (Certified Exercise Physiologist), NSCA Certified Strength and Conditioning Specialist and is a Registered Kinesiologist.

Bobbi-Jo Atchison is the Community Transition Coordinator at The Steadward Centre for Personal & Physical Achievement. She is a CSEP-CEP (Certified Exercise Physiologist); Registered Kinesiologist; and a Registered Recreational Therapist.

Karen Slater is the Associate Director of the Steadward Centre for Personal & Physical Achievement. The Steadward Centre is a disability research centre at the University of Alberta.

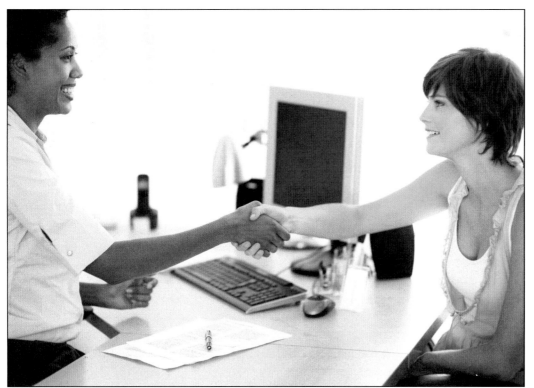

Yuri Arcurs/Shutterstock

A fitness professional may come across a wide variety of clientele throughout his/her career. Understanding the assessment process and the appropriate modifications for physical, developmental and sensory impairments will prepare the fitness professional for a range of situations in a diverse population.

The first experience a prospective client has in a fitness facility is an integral part of the appraisal process. A fitness professional should recognize that when an individual with a disability wants to begin an exercise program there may be barriers that will affect the perception of the benefits of physical activity and subsequently leading an active lifestyle. Barriers may include facility accessibility, cost, and level of knowledge and experience of fitness professionals working with individuals living with a disability.[5] Through the initial client consultation, a fitness professional should provide the individual with information about the intake process and what to expect, help ease any anxiety about joining a fitness center or changing his/her lifestyle and finally, problem solve and create and monitor realistic goals and objectives.

> **TIP:** When working with an individual to counsel or solve problems, issues may arise that are out of the scope of practice for fitness professionals. Should such an issue present itself, it is the job of the fitness professional to refer the client to appropriate health professionals.[1]

The components that should be included during the initial client consultation will be discussed throughout this section. The fitness professional may choose to go into great detail with all of these components during the initial meeting or decide that only certain aspects are necessary. What is determined will depend on the needs of the client or the questions that he/she may have during this meeting. It is always ideal to remember that the individuals coming in for the consultation will vary, as will their questions and needs. Therefore, the fitness professional will need to be flexible and conscious of the questions asked to ensure that the appropriate and necessary information is provided to the client.

Developing rapport

The main purpose when developing rapport with the client is to create a positive relationship. Establishing this relationship will generate a comfortable, trustworthy environment providing opportunity for open communication.

> **TIP:** Fitness professionals should keep in mind that communication strategies for individuals living with impairment are consistent with strategies used in communicating with individuals living without impairment. Some tips for potential modifications are made throughout this chapter.

It is very important for the fitness professional to listen attentively and utilize communication skills – both verbal and non-verbal. Non-Verbal listening skills demonstrate to the client that you are interested in what he/she has to say and that you, the fitness professional, are comfortable and at ease throughout the meeting. Knowing that the fitness professional is comfortable will often provide the client with a sense of reassurance. Additionally, recognizing the importance of these non-verbal listening skills will further enhance the relationship between the fitness professional and the client.

The following points outline key factors for non-verbal listening skills.[1, 2]

- *Eye Contact*: Establish and maintain eye contact when listening. It is preferable for the client and the fitness professional to be at eye level throughout the conversation. Dependant on the client's position the fitness professional may need to adjust their own position while being mindful of personal space. For example sitting in a chair or bending at knees while talking with someone in a wheelchair.

- *Body Language*: Always offer a handshake by way of introduction, regardless of hand and arm functioning. The fitness professional should face the client at all times.

- *Vocal Tone and Rate of Speech*: In most situations it is important to maintain regular volume and rate of speech when talking to the client. When discussing new information, it is important to speak at an appropriate pace to ensure understanding. Avoid using slang and patronizing language. For example if working with a client living with a hearing impairment, maintain volume suitable for conversation and avoid shouting as this may hinder communication.

- *Physical Space*: If possible, conversation should be approximately an arm's length away with no barriers between the client and the fitness professional. Conduct the meeting in a comfortable, well lit room – separated from the noise and activity in the fitness center.

- *Time*: Ensure that the consultation is scheduled at a time that is suitable for the client. It is important that the individual not feel rushed and has a sufficient amount of time to ask questions.

As the client and fitness professional begin to discuss the processes of beginning an exercise program, the use of active listening skills is imperative. Knowledge of these skills will enable the fitness professional to give the client time to talk; this is especially true if the individual experiences delayed speech or memory difficulties. It is important to encourage the client to discuss concerns, feelings of anxiety, or barriers that they may have while pursuing an active lifestyle. However, the fitness professional must recognize that some individuals may be eager to discuss these points, while others may be more hesitant. Tips for encouraging discussion include the following:[1]

1. Ask **open and closed ended questions** at the appropriate time. This will allow the fitness professional to obtain the necessary information specific to the intake process while also gathering information about the client's interests, likes and dislikes and previous involvement in physical activity. Open ended questions also give the fitness professional the opportunity to prompt clients to share more information. For example, asking a question like "What kind of activities interests you" will result in a more detailed answer than "Do you like basketball?"

2. As the client is talking, it is important for the fitness professional to **paraphrase or restate** what the client has said. This ensures that the fitness professional understands the point of the client's statements and can help to encourage the client to continue with their thoughts. In addition, paraphrasing reflects the fitness professional's interest in what the client is saying and can also help keep the conversation on track.

Communication strategies

When working with a client that has difficulty communicating or comprehending important details, the fitness professional may need to seek alternative communication strategies. Assistive devices such as word and picture boards and computer software can help the appraiser correspond with their client.

Often an individual will be accompanied by a guardian, assistant or other health care professional. Having an assistive individual that knows the client well during the initial client consultation can provide assistance when asking questions about current level of activity or if more complicated topics need to be discussed (*e.g.*, behavior, motivation level, supervision requirements). The fitness professional should make sure they continue to speak with the client directly. The appraiser can request and obtain permission to speak to the assistant if needed.

Pre-program screening

Collecting information on an individual's disability is essential during the pre-program screen. Through knowledge of the impairment, the fitness professional can collect more information about the commonalities and contraindications to exercise through available literature and other resources.

Each client will show differences in their abilities and level of impairment (*e.g.*, an individual with cerebral palsy may have between one to four limbs affected; differences in speech and comprehension; and mobility. Keeping the following points in mind will be helpful during the initial consultation.

- *Access to the Community* – Questions can be asked to determine whether or not an individual has participated in community activities of any kind. They will also indicate if the individual is familiar with exercising in a fitness center setting or what kind of activities they are interested in.

- *Function and Mobility* – Observation of function and mobility can provide the fitness professional with an understanding of the client's abilities. This may be helpful in guiding the fitness professional when preparing the assessment. Function and mobility are best determined during activity, the fitness professional may choose to employ a functional measurement tool to further observe mobility and function with the client.

- *Comprehension* – Depending on the individual's impairment, their level of cognition may be affected. Reduced cognitive ability can range from memory loss, to difficulty understanding, to trouble with problem solving. The fitness professional must remember that an individual's ability to perform physical activity may be indirectly affected by a cognitive disability or memory impairment. In addition, it is important to note that comprehension can be affected by time of day, fatigue, medication, pain and other secondary conditions typically associated with physical impairments.

Facility tour

Becoming accustomed to the physical space of the facility is very important. A tour of the facility, led by a staff member of the fitness center, will prove to be very beneficial to ease nerves and ensure individuals with sensory, cognitive and/or physical impairments can access the space safely and comfortably. Introducing clients to staff that will be monitoring the fitness floor establishes a point of contact for the client in the event they need assistance in the facility while they are exercising.

Clients should know the locations of the locker rooms/bathrooms and facility staff should ensure that these areas of the facility are accessible. Braille should be located under signage so that individuals with visual impairments can identify where these facilities are located.

Individuals with a visual impairment should have ample opportunity to learn the layout of the facility to increase confidence to move through the fitness facility. Giving them time to feel and understand the equipment can help reduce anxiety when starting an exercise program. Resources can be obtained from various organizations within the community to assist with this.

Assessment preparation — client

As the initial consultation comes to an end, the individual should be informed that a fitness appraisal will follow at a time agreed upon by both the fitness professional and the client. The client should know how long the fitness appraisal will take and what time to arrive at the facility. Reminders of preparation details should occur at this time so adequate planning can take place.

Some reminders may include:[1, 4]

- No vigorous exercise 6 hours prior to appraisal

- No alcohol 6 hours prior to appraisal

- No caffeine or nicotine 2 hours prior to appraisal

- No heavy meals 2 hours prior to appraisal

- Ensure all forms are filled out and returned on day of assessment

- Wear loose, comfortable clothing

They should also be informed of the testing protocols that will be administered and what the expectation will be. If the client has time to review this information it may further decrease any anxiety that comes with a fitness appraisal.[4]

Individuals with a cognitive, memory or sensory impairment should be informed about the necessary assessment preparation in a format that is easy for them to understand. Providing a written, pictorial or Braille take-home reminder for the individual is a good idea. The reminder should include preliminary instructions for the assessment as well as the date and time. This is one way to ensure the individual remembers what is required of them for his or her assessment. It is also important for the fitness professional to determine if the client is able to comprehend the take-home information. It may be best to also explain or provide the information to a family member, assistant or friend. Be sure to ask the individual what strategy is most effective for them and what level of involvement (if any) is required from a third party (family, friend or assistant).

Ensuring that the client fully understands the process is extremely important as their mood, memory, and confusion can affect the results of the assessment.[3] In some cases, performing a trial assessment with the client at the time of the consultation can assist the client in learning the necessary protocols and can help them become comfortable with the equipment, appraiser and environment.[2, 3]

Summary

The first contact between the fitness professional and client will impact the decisions each client makes when engaging in physical activity. To provide a client with the best experience when becoming active, the fitness professional should ensure that the initial consultation eases any apprehension and creates a comfortable environment. The client should have ample opportunity to become familiar with the environment they will be active in; therefore, it is important that time is left for a facility tour as well as a question and answer session. For the fitness professional, it is important to gain as much knowledge as possible about the client through the pre-program screen and discussion questions so the professional can develop a program best suited to the client's goals, abilities and needs.

References

1. Canadian Society of Exercise Physiology (2004). The Canadian physical activity, fitness & lifestyle approach (3rd ed.). Ottawa, ON: Canadian Society of Exercise Physiology.

2. Canadian Society of Exercise Physiology (2002). Inclusive fitness & lifestyle services for all disAbilities. Ottawa, ON: Canadian Society of Exercise Physiology.

3. Horvat M., Block M., & Kelly L.E. (2007). Developmental and Adapted Physical Activity Assessment. Champaign, IL: Human Kinetics

4. American College of Sports Medicine(2010). ACSM's Resource Manual for Guidelines for Exercise Testing and Prescription (6th Ed.). Baltimore, MD: Lippincott Williams & Wilkins.

5. Rimmer JH., et.al. (2004). Physical Activity Participation among persons with disabilities: Barriers and Facilitators. American Journal of Preventative Medicine,26, 419-425

CHAPTER 9

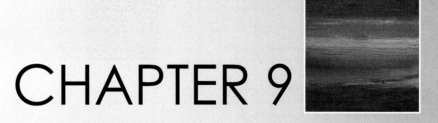

Client-Centered Goals and Objectives

By Kirsti Van Dornick, BSc. Kin.;

Bobbi-Jo Atchison, B.P.E.;

and Karen Slater, M.A.

Goal setting provides clients with the blueprint to a healthy lifestyle. Gaining a good understanding of the client's goals for physical activity is critical to developing a program and determining areas to evaluate and track progress.[2] When creating goals, including the client is extremely important, as they are the ones that will have to implement the changes to achieve the desired outcome.

As clients work to develop their own goals, they begin to work through and problem-solve ways in which these objectives will be achieved. The clients will begin to take ownership over the changes they want to see in their fitness, health, or body weight and as a result will be more inclined to work toward the potential solutions to see results.[2]

Client's goals will vary depending on their age, disability, interests and health along with other variables. Fitness professionals must be prepared to address objectives ranging from basic activities of daily living — for example carrying groceries or reaching the top shelf of their cupboards to engaging in sports at a high competition level, for example Paralympics or Special Olympics. Regardless of the goal set out by the client, the fitness professional should take the necessary steps to incorporate each objective into the physical activity plan.

The fitness professional may also experience a client that describes a goal that is beyond their scope of practice. Fitness professionals should be prepared to refer their client where necessary or consult other professionals as needed.

When working with an individual with a disability, there are often a number of health professionals providing service to the client. Examples of individuals involved in the client's team of professionals may include doctors, physiotherapists, occupational therapists, clinical exercise physiologists, nutritionists and psychologists. Fitness professionals should align exercise prescriptions with the desired outcomes of the other professionals[3] while ensuring that the client's voice is heard. An exercise program created solely on the requests of health professionals can create a sense of "dependence" or "disempowerment" for the client[2] and therefore decrease the likelihood of continuing with the fitness program. Creating a program that includes input directly from the client along with exercises recommended by health professionals will create balance and still give the client ownership over their decisions to engage in physical activity.

Individuals with cognitive disabilities may have difficulty articulating their goals; however fitness professionals should encourage and support all individuals to make decisions about their exercise program.

A variety of tools and principles are used to develop goals, however one of the most basic tools – the SMART Principle – covers the variables to set and achieve goals.

- Specific: Ensuring that the goal is specific will allow the fitness professional to develop a program with a focus in areas the client wishes to improve.

- Measurable: There should always be a way to measure the desired outcome. Gauging change at set intervals over the course of the program will allow the fitness professional to make necessary changes to the program if the benchmark goals are not being met, as well as motivate the client to continue their fitness program when improvements are evident.

- Attainable: Goals should be set to be achieved. Start with small goals and

Figure 1. SMART Principle goal setting questionnaire.[1]

When setting goals, play it SMART. Goals should be Specific, Measurable, Attainable, Realistic, and have a Time

frame for completion.

Goals and Action Steps   **Time Frame**

Goal #1 _____   _____

Action Steps

1.   _____   _____

2.   _____   _____

3.   _____   _____

Goal #2 _____   _____

Action Steps

1.   _____   _____

2.   _____   _____

3.   _____   _____

Goal #3 _____   _____

Action Steps

1.   _____   _____

2.   _____   _____

3.   _____   _____

Success Indicators

1. _____

2. _____

3. _____

4. _____

5. _____

Date for next appraisal   _____

Source: *Canadian Physical Activity, Fitness & Lifestyle Approach: CSEP-Health & Fitness Program's Appraisal and Counselling Strategy,* 3rd edition. © 2003. Reprinted with permission from the Canadian Society of Exercise Physiology.

work from there. As the client begins to reach the benchmarks they have set for themselves it will be more probable they will adhere to their program.

- **Realistic:** It is important to ensure that the goal an individual is setting is realistic. It is possible, that as a fitness professional, you may encounter situations in which a person has an idea of what they want to achieve; yet that idea or goal may be improbable. As a result, the fitness professional may need to redirect and break the goal down into achievable components.

- **Time-orientated:** Having a time-line for a goal keeps individuals accountable for the results they have desire to achieve. Ensuring the timeline is within reason is very important to prevent frustration as it is not uncommon for individuals to plateau after rehabilitation.

Figure 1 demonstrates an example of strategic goal planning that can be used with clients.

Summary

It is critical to ensure that the client has input on the goals that will guide their exercise program. Treatment plans designed for the client through other health care professionals should be considered as well, but the focus should be on what the client wants to achieve through exercise. Tools such as the SMART principle goal setting questionnaire assist in the goal setting process – as it gives the client a visual reminder of their goal and the time-line to achieve it. It is very important for the fitness professional to work closely with the client to ensure that the goals are realistic and attainable to increase the likelihood the client will achieve the desired outcome. Start small, and gradually build up to bigger tasks. Maintaining client motivation through achievable goals, and reasonable benchmarks will increase the likelihood the client will continue to be active.

References

1. Canadian Society of Exercise Physiology (2004). The Canadian physical activity, fitness & lifestyle approach (3rd ed.). Ottawa, ON: Canadian Society of Exercise Physiology.

2. Canadian Society of Exercise Physiology (2002). Inclusive fitness & lifestyle services for all disAbilities. Ottawa, ON: Canadian Society of Exercise Physiology.

3. American College of Sports Medicine(2010). ACSM's Resource Manual for Guidelines for Exercise Testing and Prescription (6th Ed.). Baltimore, MD: Lippincott Williams & Wilkins.

CHAPTER 10

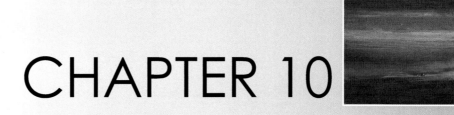

Screening, Risk Assessment, and Red Flags

By Bobbi-Jo Atchison, B.P.E.;

Kirsti Van Dornick, BSc. Kin.;

and Karen Slater, M.A.

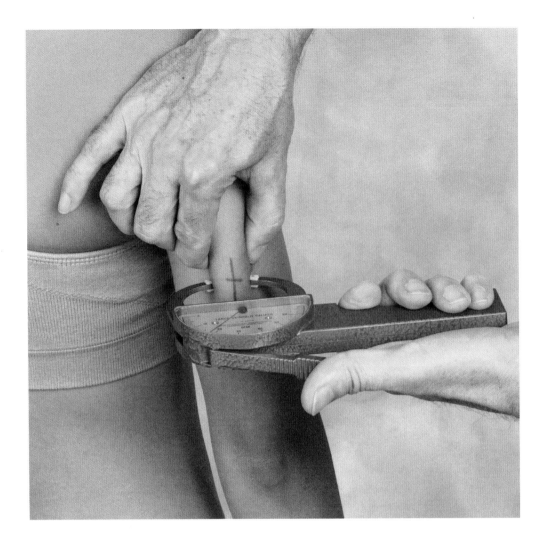

Physical activity for people experiencing disability is considered to be beneficial. Taking into consideration that many individuals with a disability lead a sedentary lifestyle, there is an increased likelihood that they will acquire secondary conditions that will be detrimental to their health and decrease their quality of life. Common secondary conditions associated with a sedentary lifestyle include but are not limited to coronary heart disease, Type 2 diabetes, and obesity. Risks associated with physical activity for persons with a disability are also prevalent and can often present themselves to individuals beginning an active lifestyle. To ensure that the most appropriate program is being provided to the client, a proper screening and risk assessment must be completed.

Screening

New clients should be filling out a series of forms that will be kept on file and will act as a reference to fitness professionals when information is required. Registration forms should include general information such as name, address, telephone numbers, medical information as well as more detailed information on medications, allergies and any emergency health conditions that the individual may be prone to under certain environmental conditions for example, seizures. The fitness professional should ensure that they understand the information provided through the registration form – such as the purpose and side effects of certain medications. It is important for the registration form to include questions about medical history as well as other risk factors that may require medical clearance prior to exercise. Upon arrival, the fitness professional should determine whether assessment preparation has taken place. If preliminary instructions have not been adhered to, the fitness professional has the ability to postpone the assessment accordingly.

Knowledge of the client's medical history will be a good indication of whether the client will need medical evaluation prior to beginning the exercise program. If the individual has experienced a heart attack in the past, has abnormal rhythm, or a congenital heart condition, then it is best to ensure that they are healthy enough to start exercising by requesting consent from their doctor. Generally, such conditions will be identified through the completion of the Physical Activity Readiness Questionnaire (PAR-Q).

The PAR-Q is valid for anyone 15- to 69-years-old of both genders and must be completed prior to assessment. This tool should be explained carefully, as clients with positive responses to the questions will need to speak to their doctor and have a PARmed – X form completed before the assessment date. A PARmed-X form must be completed if the individual is over 69 years of age. It is important that the fitness professional does not attempt to diagnose "yes" responses; however, further clarification to certain questions may be provided to ensure that questions are answered appropriately. For example, dizziness is defined as light headedness usually associated with the sensation or feeling of instability.[1] Another term used in the PAR-Q is "Heart Condition" which includes heart attack, angina, congenital heart disease, heart valve disease, congestive heart failure, edema and the use of heart medications. It is also a best practice to include any kind of cardiopulmonary surgery under this area.[1]

Despite the outcome on the PAR-Q questionnaire, medical clearance can still be obtained to collect more information specific to the individual's impairment that will help guide fitness professionals with limited experience in the area of adapted physical activity. If the fitness professional is unfamiliar with the impairment or requires more information about the client prior to assessment, it is recommended they have their client's doctor complete the PARmed-X.

A waiver and informed consent must be completed in addition to the PAR-Q. Waivers are signed statements relinquishing some level of right. Risks that are present when engaging in activity are listed in this form — covering the fitness professional of liability in the event of an accident. A waiver does not excuse irresponsibility or negligence – so it must be ensured that best practice is always used. A consent form provides information about what kind of activity will be engaged during the fitness appraisal. Youth must have a parent or guardian's signature and a witness other than the fitness professional must sign off. It is important to note that the informed consent is not a legally binding document.

Adults with a cognitive impairment are legally able to give consent in the same manner as other adults. However, the fitness professional may request another form be signed and filled out by a caregiver or guardian if there is concern that the individual does not understand the concepts covered in the consent form.[2] To ensure the client is treated with dignity at all times, permission should be sought from the client prior to seeking third party assistance. When discussing the activities that will be performed at the time of the fitness appraisal, it is important for the fitness professional to ensure that they are using terms that the client can understand. Allowing time for comprehension will prevent misunderstandings as to what is expected in the fitness assessment.

> **TIP:** In order for the PAR-Q consent and waiver forms to be valid the client must be of legal age, comprehend the importance and relevance of risks, give voluntary consent, and have a witness of legal age.

If required, the fitness professional should seek out different formats for forms, such as Braille, audio or email that will be useful if the individual has a visual impairment. Once forms are distributed, the client should be reminded to have all forms completed at the time of the assessment. It is beneficial to have the PAR-Q completed prior to the assessment to allow time to visit the doctor in the event the PAR-med-X needs to be filled out.

Once all forms are screened by the fitness professional for red flags or other concerns then further observations or areas that may be risk factors also should be addressed. Some general risk factors may include age, sedentary lifestyle, high cholesterol, smoking, hypertension and family history. When discussing the client's medical history, it will also be important to note any past musculoskeletal injuries that may limit the individual's performance.

While the PAR-Q and PARmed-X forms provide essential information there are often screening concerns that are missed. It is vital to communicate with and observe your client to ensure you are aware of the following potential red flags or contraindications that may arise during your initial assessment:

1. Fatigue: Fatigue can be a symptom associated with certain medical conditions and physical impairments. It is common for individuals to feel more fatigued at certain times of the day. If your client feels they have the most energy in the morning and prefers to do much of their daily tasks at this time, scheduling a morning assessment would be optimal. On the other hand, if your client has difficulty getting up in the morning, an afternoon or evening assessment time may be best. By working with your clients fatigue schedule rather than against it, you will receive more optimal results from the assessment. Individuals with the following conditions may be more likely to experience fatigue: multiple sclerosis, fibromyalgia, chronic fatigue syndrome and post polio.

2. Temperature: Certain types of physical impairments can affect an individual's ability to control temperature. For example, individuals with spinal cord injury have the inability to produce sweat below the level of injury, affecting their capability to naturally cool their body when performing moderate to high intensity exercise. Individuals with multiple sclerosis also commonly experience thermosensitivity. To ensure proper body cooling, allow for adequate hydration and rest periods to keep core temperatures from climbing. Extra fans or cooling devices will further prevent overheating.

3. Medications: Medications can often affect appraisal results and in some cases may require postponing the assessment until further notice. Familiarizing yourself with the medications your client is currently taking prior to the assessment will assist you in understanding the physiological responses that the client may experience. For example, if your client is taking a beta blocker, they may have decreased heart rate and blood pressure both at rest and during their exercise.[4,6] With knowledge of their medications and the associated side effects, you will be able to better incorporate tools, such as a rate of perceived exertion scale, to assist you in performing the most effective testing protocol, or understanding when a test cannot be performed.

4. Lower Extremity Swelling: Edema or swelling of the feet, ankles or legs can be a serious sign of poor circulation, deep vein thrombosis, or heart and organ failure.[5] Lower extremity swelling can, however, also be caused by prolonged sitting and standing or certain medications. If your client is experiencing a sudden onset of fluid buildup in their lower extremities, encourage them to see their doctor and postpone assessment until you receive written approval or a PARmed-X from a medical professional.

5. Blood Glucose: Assessing blood glucose levels may be necessary when working with a client who has diabetes or a history of low blood sugars. Typical measures of fasting blood glucose range from 60 – 99 mg/dL. Impaired fasting glucose ranges from 100 – 125 mg/dL. If glucose levels are impaired, ask the client to wait 10 to 15 minutes and then request that they check their blood glucose level again to make sure it is in the desired range.[3]

6. Difficulty Breathing at Rest: If client is observed to have difficulty breathing at rest, encourage them to see their doctor and postpone assessment until you receive written approval or a PARmed-X from a medical professional.

7. Pregnancy: if your client is pregnant, a fitness assessment and program can be prescribed. It is important to have the participant request that a PARmed-X for Pregnancy be filled out by a medical professional.

Risk Assessment

Prior to performing a fitness appraisal, a risk assessment must be initiated. Obtaining resting heart rate, blood pressure, along with height and weight measurements can educate the fitness professional of current or potential red flags that may arise. The risk assessment will also give the fitness professional a clear indication of a client's current health status with relation to normative values of heart rate, blood pressure and Body Mass Index. Heart rate and blood pressure measurement criteria are consistent across individuals with and without a disability.

Resting heart rate measurement

Measuring resting heart rate is an important step in screening for potential risks and ensuring that a client can safely engage in all aspects of the fitness appraisal. A person's resting heart rate can be influenced by several factors including anxiety, caffeine, nicotine, medication and the type of activity they are engaged in. To ensure accuracy, it is important to be aware of current medications and that the client follows all preliminary instructions prior to an appointment.

Equipment: Stop-watch or Heart Rate Monitor

Procedure: Have client rest in a comfortable seated position for approximately five minutes. A brief relaxation period can assist in easing assessment anxiety and help to reduce heart rate to resting levels for a more accurate reading. If possible, the client should be seated upright and have both feet flat on the floor or wheelchair foot plates. The heart rate can be measured manually using a 15 second count (multiplied by four) by applying gentle pressure with your index and middle finger to the radial or carotid artery.[1] For clients who experience asymmetrical weakness, taking their heart rate on the stronger or functional side will yield more accurate results.

If the resting heart rate is above 100 beats per minute (bpm), have your client sit for an additional 5 minutes and re-test. If their heart rate continues to be above 100 bpm they should not be permitted to perform the aerobic or musculoskeletal portion of the assessment. Recommend that the client discuss heart rate results with their physician. Anthropometric measurements can still be completed.

TIP: Heart rate measurement for individuals with poor circulation can be difficult to determine manually as palpation can be complicated. Using a wrist watch heart rate monitor *without* the chest strap can ensure you get a near accurate reading before continuing with your assessment. Chest straps are not recommended as they can be difficult to put on — causing anxiety and requiring client to disrobe. Chest straps are also difficult to keep in place on a person's chest if they have poor posture or sit in a wheelchair that does not allow them to maintain a straight posture.

Resting blood pressure measurement

Similar to resting heart rate, resting blood pressure must be taken as a precautionary step and ensure that the participant can safely engage in all aspects of the fitness appraisal. Blood pressure can be influenced by many factors including anxiety, caffeine, nicotine and medications. Once again, to ensure accuracy, it is important to be aware of current medications and that the client follows all preliminary instructions prior to appointment.

Equipment: Chair with back and arm supports, stethoscope, sphygmomanometer with appropriate sized cuff

Procedure: While seated upright in a comfortable chair with arm supported at heart level, apply appropriate sized cuff to participant's left arm. Wrap cuff smoothly and firmly around arm aligning with brachial artery, with the lower margin two or three centimeters above antecubital space. Place stethoscope over brachial artery and inflate cuff to 20 mmHg above first Korottkoff sound and release pressure at a rate of 2 – 5 mm-per-second.[5]

If the client experiences significant impairment on the left side due to contractures, muscle weakness or paralysis, the cuff should be applied to client's right arm. If you are unable to measure blood pressure on either arm due to amputations or severe contractures, blood pressure can be taken using the popliteal fossa artery in the upper leg. It is important to note that systolic pressure may be 20 to 30 mmHg higher in the thigh than that of the arm.[2]

> **TIP:** For fitness testing, there are generally three different cuff sizes to choose from when taking blood pressure measurements, a pediatric cuff for youth or small adults (7- to 10 ¾ inches), an adult cuff (9.5- to 14 ¼ inches) and a large adult cuff (13- to 19 ½ inches) for bariatric participants. Adult thigh cuffs (18- to 26 inches) are also available if the large adult cuff does not fit.

If resting blood pressure is above 160/100 mmHg have client rest five minutes and re-test. If blood pressure remains over 160/100 mmHg client should not be permitted to perform the aerobic testing and musculoskeletal testing. Recommend that the client discuss blood pressure results with their physician.

Anthropometric measurements can still be completed.

> **TIP:** If client has latex allergies, you may need to use a latex free cuff to prevent an allergic reaction. Latex allergies are common in persons with spina bifida or individuals who have undergone frequent surgeries.

Weight and height measurements

Gathering weight and height measurements is an important aspect of the risk assessment as it provides the fitness professional a means to calculate normative measurements such as Body Mass Index (BMI). Calculating one's BMI assists in determining if a person is within a 'healthy' zone or a 'high risk' zone. See description of *Body Mass Index* below for more information.

When assessing weight and height of an individual with a disability, the fitness professional can usually follow standard protocol. In many cases however, minor adjustments and modifications will need to be made in order to gather accurate information. Some of these circumstances may include a client who is unable to balance without assistance or those who have experienced limb loss or lower body paralysis.

Weight measurement

Equipment. Standard Scale or Chair Scale or Wheelchair Scale

Procedure:

- Standard Scale: Ensure scale is on a flat surface and is calibrated properly. If client is able to stand upright without leaning heavily on a mobility aid, it is possible to weigh them on a standard scale. If a mobility aid is needed, such as a cane, ankle foot orthotic or leg brace, the aid must be measured separately and subtracted from the total weight of client: *(mobility aid + client) – (mobility aid) = Total Weight.*
- Chair Scale: Ensure scale is on a flat surface and is calibrated properly. If possible, have client remove footwear and any excess clothing or equipment such as a transfer belt. If this is not possible, the fitness professional must record this modification. Have the client transfer into chair, measure weight accordingly.
- Wheelchair Scale: Ensure scale is on a flat surface and is calibrated properly. If possible have client remove any excess baggage, clothing or oxygen tank from chair. Have the client transfer out of chair onto a comfortable area. Measure chair only and record measurement, fitness professional must indicate if there is any excess baggage or clothing that was unable to be removed. Have client transfer back into chair and measure both chair and client together. Record measurement and calculate: *(chair + client) – (chair only) = Total Weight.*

TIP: If unsafe to transfer participant out of chair, chair weight can be collected from manufacturer or through the family physician.

Height measurement

Equipment: Measuring tape, ruler, water soluble marker, wall or mat or wide bench

Procedure:

- Standing Height: Without footwear (if possible), have the client stand as tall as possible, with feet slightly apart for balance.[4] If the person is able to keep heals in contact with wall, have them do so. The fitness professional must record modifications made in full detail including but not limited to, flexion in hip, distance heels are away from wall, footwear worn and/or mobility aid or prosthetic device if used. Mark measurement on wall, once client has moved and is seated safely, measure the distance from the floor to the mark on the wall.
- Supine Height: For individuals unable to weight bear or stand straight due to contractures, muscle weakness or paralysis, height measurement can be taken lying down on a raised bench or mat.[4] Place one end of mat or bench against wall. Without footwear (if possible), have client lie supine with feet against wall, lying as straight as possible. To measure, have participant stretch as tall as possible against the mat (gentle traction may be required in some cases).[4] This may take more than one professional dependent on the level of contractures or spasticity the client may experience. Mark a meas-

urement using a ruler and marker on bench or mat. Once the client has moved and is safely seated, measure distance between wall and mark on bench or mat.[4]

TIP: If you are unable to correctly measure height of the participant in the upright or supine position then the measurement also can be taken by measuring the extended arm length of client. Measurements are taken from tip of middle finger on laterally extended right arm across chest to tip of middle finger on extended left arm.

Body mass index

While Body Mass Index (BMI) can be easily assessed with a simple calculation of weight and height (kg/m2) of an individual, for some people with physical impairments the numbers may not reveal valid and accurate results. When calculating and revealing the results of BMI for your client, it is important to keep the following in mind. How did you measure their weight? Do they have atrophied limbs or amputations? How did you measure their height? Do they have scoliosis or a form of spinal degeneration? Did you measure with prosthetics? What these questions tell us is that the reliability of the measurement results may not be accurate enough to get a true Body Mass Index. For example, an individual with an amputated leg may weigh less and fall within a 'healthy' BMI despite excess adipose tissue on their body. This does not mean that you cannot use BMI to assist you, but it is important to think critically when using this protocol. Inform your client of any areas that may disrupt the validity and reliability of this tool.

Red Flags and Contraindications

As with any fitness appraisal, there are potential risks to performing physical fitness assessments. More common occurrences can include, but are not limited to: autonomic dysreflexia (AD), seizures, allergic reactions, mood altercations, and contractures. Table 1 explains each condition and provides an action plan to prevent or administer assistance if needed.

Summary

Conducting accurate preliminary screening, observation and risk assessment on each client before beginning the cardiovascular and musculoskeletal testing component of an assessment is a key factor to ensuring a safe and comfortable environment for the client. Thorough screening will provide the fitness professional with enough information to

Table 1. Contraindications to Exercise.

CONDITION	WHAT IS IT?	HOW TO PREVENT IT?	ADMINISTERED ASSISTANCE
Autonomic Dysreflexia (AD)	A sudden onset of physiological responses that include hypertension, bradycardia, headache and sweating caused by overstimulation of the autonomic nervous system.[6] Most common in persons with a spinal cord injury.	Ensure bladder is empty and any form of painful stimuli is not affecting individual (pressure sore, pinching, burning or rubbing of paralyzed limbs)	If AD is present, remove stimulus immediately. If symptoms persist contact emergency assistance as stated through your emergency action plan.
Seizures	Several forms including grand mal, petite mal and febrile, can cause loss of consciousness, bladder function, convulsions and confusion. Most common in persons with epilepsy, stroke or brain injury	Be familiar with clients seizure history, ensure medications are taken if needed, understand environmental triggers	Ensure participant is in a safe position and not harming themselves or others, contact emergency assistance as stated through your emergency action plan
Allergic Reactions	Latex allergies can be common in persons with spina bifida	Be familiar with client's allergy history. Ensure equipment used during assessment is latex free (Including medicine balls, tubing, resistance bands, blood pressure cuffs)	If participant has an allergic reaction – remove stimulus immediately. If symptoms continue contact emergency assistance as stated through your emergency action plan
Mood Outburst	Participant may feel angry, upset or highly confused, may be common in persons with brain injury or dementia	Ensure participant has full understanding of each task asked of them, remain calm at all times	Ensure participant is not harming themselves or others. Stop assessment and remove individual from environment and stimulus that may be causing reaction
Contracture	A permanent shortening of muscle, tendon or ligament. Most typically found in ankle, knee, hips, elbow and wrist joints. May be common in individuals with cerebral palsy or stroke.t	Stretching and range of motion can reduce the prevalence	Be familiar with the location and severity of the contracture. Do not force the affected limb(s) through range of motion. Choice of suitable exercise and equipment options will optimize workout and comfort

know if further medical clearance is needed from a client's physician. The initial screening, observation and risk assessment will also ensure the fitness professional is aware of any potential red flags and confirms that the full fitness appraisal can be performed.

References

1. Canadian Society of Exercise Physiology (2004). The Canadian physical activity, fitness & lifestyle approach (3rd ed.). Ottawa, ON: Canadian Society of Exercise Physiology.

2. Canadian Society of Exercise Physiology (2002). Inclusive fitness & lifestyle services for all disAbilities. Ottawa, ON: Canadian Society of Exercise Physiology.

3. American College of Sport Medicine (2013). ACSM's Guidelines for Exercise Testing and Prescription (9th Edition). Philladelphia PA: Lippincott Williams & Wilkins.

4. Rick Hansen Centre (1993). Fitness assessment manual (3rd ed.). Edmonton, AB: Rick Hansen Centre.

5. American College of Sports Medicine (2010). ACSM's Guidelines for Exercise Testing and Prescription (8th Edition). Philladelphia PA: Lippincott Williams & Wilkins.

6. Durstine L. J. & Moore G. E. (2003). ACSM's Exercise management for persons with chronic diseases and disabilities (2nd ed.). Champaign, IL: Human Kinetics.

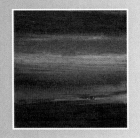

CHAPTER 11

Health, Physical Fitness, and Functional Assessments

By Bobbi-Jo Atchison, B.P.E.;
Kirsti Van Dornick, BSc. Kin.;
and Karen Slater, M.A.

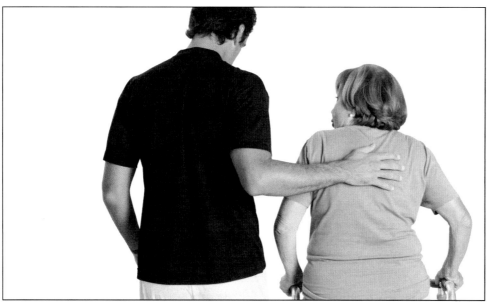
Bigstock

When performing a fitness appraisal, it is important to understand the difference between normative referenced assessments and criterion referenced assessments. Normative referenced assessments, like those intended for apparently fit individuals, compares a person's performance against norms of participants their age range and gender. Criterion referenced assessments, similar to those performed on persons with a disability compare a person's performance to a preferred level of completion.[1]

It is possible to use normative referenced criteria on certain tasks of an assessment for individuals with disabilities. However, once an assessment is modified it is no longer appropriate to use normative comparisons. For this reason, it is more common to use a criterion referenced appraisal for individuals who are unable to complete the normative referenced protocol.

This raises a question: If an inclusive fitness trainer is unable to collect normative data from an assessment, then why assess? Performing fitness assessments on persons with a disability are important for many reasons. Assessments provide the fitness professional with ample opportunity to screen for potential red flags or contraindications specific to their client. This also is a good time to observe your participants function and mobility within the exercise environment, for example, ability to transfer on and off equipment or grip objects such as free weights and equipment handles. Furthermore, the fitness professional will have the opportunity to gather additional information in order to develop the fitness program that will best meet the client's individualized goals and abilities.

When assessing an individual with a cognitive or learning impairment the fitness professional may be required to break tasks into smaller steps to ensure the participant has a full understanding of the actions required. No matter what a client's abilities are, each test should be re-explained in full detail once an assessment task is ready. In some cases, it may be required to take the participant through a practice assessment prior to performing the actual assessment.[2] This will provide less anxiety and better understanding for the client, while providing the fitness professional with a clear understanding of when and where verbal, physical or written cueing may be needed.

Assessment Preparation for Fitness Professionals

Equipment choice is vital when preparing an assessment for a person with a disability. Typical fitness testing equipment is not always suitable for persons with mobility impairments or balance and coordination difficulties. For example, in many cases, using stairs to perform a cardiovascular test will not be appropriate when an individual is in a wheelchair or does not have proper strength and/or balance to perform a standard step test.

Understanding a person's abilities will assist the fitness professional in choosing the best suited equipment for fitness testing. Standard equipment options are available; however, in many cases further adaptations are needed. Table 1 shows equipment options available for testing cardiovascular endurance, muscular strength and muscular endurance for persons with mobility impairments.

Table 1. Equipment options for fitness testing

Cardiovascular		Musculoskeletal	
Standard	Modified	Standard	Modified
Monark Ergometer	Step through recumbent ergometer or arm ergometer	Hand dynamometer	Finger web
Standard Treadmill	Treadmill with long hand rails and low step up	Vertex	Weight machines/Medicine Balls
Indoor Track	Arm ergometer	Bench Press	Free weights/Velcro weights/Tubing and bands
Steps	Steps with hand rails	Floor Mat	Wide bench / raised mat
Rowing ergometer	Rowing ergometer without seat		

Alternate Planning

Based on information collected through a client consultation, the fitness professional should have an idea of the client's abilities when choosing an appropriate assessment protocol. At times, the participant's perceived abilities may not match their actual capabilities during exercise. An alternate plan of action will allow the fitness professional to be well prepared if the initial plan is unsuccessful. For example, if assessing muscular endurance of a client in a wheelchair, the fitness professional may wish to do a bench press with them. What is the next step if a client is unable to transfer to the narrow bench provided? Often, transferring for wheelchair users can be extremely difficult due to the demands placed on the upper body and core stabilizer muscles. Because muscles of the upper body are prone to overuse injuries due to prolonged wheelchair use, muscular fatigue and pain can often accompany individuals who make difficult transfers onto constricted platforms. Having an alternate plan will help an inclusive fitness trainer be prepared for several different possibilities prior to an assessment.

Plan A	Alternate Plan
Bench Press	Bench Press on wide bench or
	Bench Press on raised Mat or
	Chest Press with Free Weights, Body Bars or Machine

By preparing for best and worst case scenarios, a trainer can maintain professionalism, client confidence, and perform a proficient assessment.

Test Termination

Test termination criteria for persons with disabilities follows the same guidelines as traditional test termination criteria; however, it is important to understand that there are often additional reasons for test termination with this population. Not only are persons with a disability more likely to have secondary health conditions, they are commonly on medications that may affect their performance and physiological response to exercise. There is also an increased probability that an individual with a memory or cognitive impairment may have difficulty understanding processes or fail to remember a process midway through a required task. It is of utmost importance to determine test termination criteria prior to your assessment. See Table 2 for examples of test termination criteria.[3]

Table 2. Test termination criteria

Test Termination Criteria
Requirements of test have been achieved
Maximum HR reached
Angina / Chest Pain
Onset of lightheadedness or dizziness
BP drops more than 10 mmHg
Excessively high BP (250/115)
Client asks for test to be terminated
Client appears confused or agitated
Volitional fatigue, pain or spasms do not allow for continuous proper technique
Client experiences symptoms of Autonomic Dysreflexia
Changes in vision
Difficulty breathing during testing

Testing Protocol

Anthropometric Measurements

Body composition measurement is a great way to gain a better understanding of your client's physical proportions and potential areas of improvement. There is a variety of anthropometric measurement tools used to assess apparently healthy populations. Girth measurements, skin folds, hydrostatic weighing, Bod Pod and Bioelectrical Impedance Analysis are a few examples. With a variety of different tools available on the market today to test one's body composition, it is important for the assessor to research what would work best and yield the most accurate results for their client.

Anthropometric measurements often require an appraiser to get physically up close to the client or can sometimes require the individual to be placed into an uncomfortable position for a period of time. Because of this, anthropometric measurements can often be intimidating or embarrassing for participants who lead sedentary lifestyles or have a lack of understanding about the testing protocols. It is vital to fully explain testing protocol and obtain the participant's permission before administering testing procedures.

> **TIP:** When conducting anthropometric measurements such as girth measurements and skin folds on a client it is important to measure only those sites where functional muscle exists.[4]

Girth measurements

For persons who have asymmetrical muscle development, girth measurements should be taken on both sides of the body. For clients who experience paralysis, girth measurements should only focus on areas of the body where functional muscle exists.[4]

Equipment: Measuring Tape and water soluble marker
Procedures: Girth sites may include chest, biceps, waist, hips, thigh and calf.

> **TIP:** A client may sit or stand depending on abilities and preferences unless otherwise stated below.

- Chest: Arms should be relaxed beside body, measure mid-sternum at the end of normal expiration.[4]
- Biceps: Arm should be relaxed and extended fully at side, measure midway between acromion and tip of elbow.[4]
- Waist: Measure 3 cm above the navel or between the bottom of the rib cage and the top of the iliac crest.[4]

> **TIP:** Measuring waist circumference on an individual in a seated position can be difficult. This is due to the posture that often accompanies individuals with limited abdominal function or long-time wheelchair use and, therefore, can yield invalid results. If possible, have the client lift and hold themselves off their chair using armrests for support. This position will allow their trunk to be extended for a more accurate measurement. If this is not possible, the client can lie on a

raised mat or bench and measurements can be taken. The appraiser must record any modifications.[4]

- Hips: Should only be performed on clients who have the ability to engage in lower body activities while weight bearing.[4] The client should stand with feet slightly apart and weight distributed as evenly as possible, a balance aid may be used if needed. Measure the maximum girth over buttocks.
- Thigh: Should only be performed on clients who have the ability to engage in lower body activities while weight bearing. Participant should stand with feet shoulder width apart and distribute weight as evenly as possible; a balance aid may be used if needed. Measurement can be taken 1 cm below the gluteal line.[4]
- Calf: Should only be performed on clients who have the ability to engage in lower body activities while weight bearing. Participant should stand with feet shoulder width apart and distribute weight as evenly as possible; a balance aid may be used if needed. Measurements should be taken at the point of maximum girth.[4]

Skinfold measurement

Skinfold measurement can be performed on persons with a disability, but considerations and adaptations may be required. While skinfold testing is generally measured on the right side of the body, if an individual experiences weakness or paralysis on this side, measurements should be taken on their left side. If the individual experiences lower body paralysis, measurement should not be taken, as the distinction between adipose tissue and paralyzed muscle can be difficult to measure and result in inaccurate measurements.[4]

Equipment: High quality calipers and water soluble marker

Procedure: Skinfold sites may include triceps, biceps, subscapular, iliac crest and medial calf

- Triceps: Client may sit or stand depending on abilities and preference. With arm extended comfortably at side and palm facing leg or chair, measure midway between acromion and tip of elbow.[5]
- Biceps: Client may sit or stand depending on abilities and preference. With arm extended comfortably at side and palm facing forward, measure at midpoint through bicep belly at same level as tricep measurement.[5]
- Subscapular: It is optimal for a client to stand with arms extended comfortably at side with palms facing body. If client is unable to stand and can sit in a wheelchair or stationary chair with a low backing, measurements can be taken. Measure 1 cm below the inferior angle of the scapula at an angle 45 degrees to the spine.[5]
- Iliac Crest: Client must stand for accurate results, a mobility aid may be used as long as participant is able to stand erect during measurement. Have client elevate elbow to shoulder height, preferably in a horizontal position. Skinfold is measured 3 cm above the crest of the ilium at the midline point of the body.[5]
- Medial Calf: Client must stand for accurate results, a mobility aid may be

used with no limitation to weight bearing on required aid. Have client place relaxed foot onto a raised flat object that allows for their knee to be bent at a 90 degree angle. Measurement is taken on inside of calf at the level of maximum girth.[5]

Additional methods of assessing body composition

Bioelectrical Impedance Analysis, Bod Pod, air displacement, plethysmography and hydrostatic weighing are examples of additional methods of testing body composition. These tools often require more equipment, training and each have their advantages and disadvantages. Each method should be researched properly on their effectiveness and appropriateness for the prospective client's cognitive and physical abilities.

Cardiovascular testing

Cardiovascular fitness testing allows the fitness professional to calculate the ability of their client to perform dynamic exercise at moderate to high intensities, utilizing large muscle groups for prolonged periods.[3] The common non-clinical test performed on able-bodied populations is the Step Test. While this test does an effective job of assessing maximal oxygen intake with limited equipment and set up, it is not always appropriate for individuals with mobility, visual, balance or cognitive impairments. See Table 3 for a list of tests available, along with adaptations and recommendations for a variety of abilities. Some individuals may have difficulty with hand placement on equipment due to limited grip strength, or foot placement on cycle ergometer due to drop foot or paralysis. To accommodate, hand ties or foot straps can be used while maintaining the reliability of the testing protocol. See figure 1 and figure 2 for examples of these adaptations.

Figure 1. Example of tensor bandage used to aid with grip strength on arm ergometer.

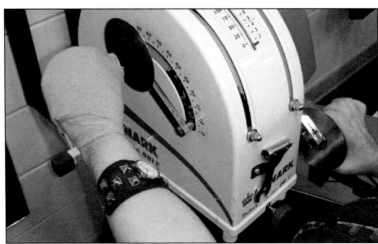

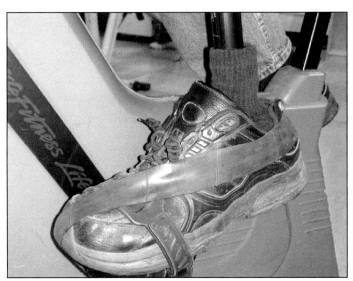

Figure 2.
Example of inner
tube strap used to
keep placement of
foot in pedal.

Table 3. Cardiovascular endurance testing

Test Options	Sub Maximal Tests Available	Equipment Options	Adaptations & Recommendations
Ambulatory	Rockport	Treadmill or 200 meter track	Use of mobility aid or treadmill with hand rails for balance
	Modified 12 Minute or 6 Minute Walk	Treadmill or 200 meter track	Use of mobility aid or treadmill with hand rails for balance
	Step Test	Double steps or single step	Steps with hand rails for balance Visual metronome to time steps for clients with hearing impairments Foot placement pads for clients with memory impairments
Seated	Modified Astrand	Cycle ergometer	Foot straps to assist foot placement, decrease RPM if needed
	YMCA	Cycle ergometer	Foot straps to assist foot placement, decrease RPM
	PWC 150	Cycle ergometer	Foot straps to assist foot placement, decrease RPM if needed
Upper Body	Modified Astrand	Arm ergometer	Hand ties to assist limited grip strength
	12 min test	200 meter track	Standard or sport wheelchair
	MACAFT	Arm ergometer	Hand ties to assist limited grip strength

The participant's maximum heart rate should be calculated prior to a cardiovascular test and noted on the assessment forms. Maximum heart rate can be calculated using 220 – age = maximum heart rate. As mentioned earlier in this chapter, it is possible for a person's heart rate to vary depending on several different factors, in turn, distorting results. For example, performing a test on an arm ergometer produces a maximal heart rate response 10 bpm less than leg exercise.[7] Because heart rate does not always portray the physiological results expected, it is important to use additional tools to monitor intensity of the activity.

> **TIP:** Maximum heart rate can be different for some individuals based on their level of impairment. For example: Individuals with developmental disabilities will often have a maximum heart rate 8 – 20% lower than able–bodied populations.[6]

Additional Methods for Monitoring Intensity

The Borg Scale's Rating of Perceived Exertion (RPE) uses a number system to describe how hard one perceives they are working. This quick and easy tool is highly recommended when working with individuals with impairments. It allows the fitness professional to gain a better idea as to the level of work a client perceives or feels that they are performing. This can often assist the appraiser to better understand what level of intensity their client is working, even if their heart rate levels have not reached the desired test levels.

- Advantages: requires limited tools, two different tools to choose from (6 – 20 scale and 0 – 10 scale), print material easily accessed.
- Disadvantages: RPE 6 – 20 scale can be difficult to understand, it is common for participants to rate their exertions levels higher or lower than what they are physiologically presenting (*i.e.,* sweating, red face, decreased ability to perform task at hand).

> **TIP:** If working with someone who has a cognitive or memory impairment, the 0 -10 scales may be easier to comprehend than the original 6 – 20 Borg Scale. Holding a large written scale, or providing a picture scale may also be helpful.

The Talk Test is another method used to easily assess intensity levels of exercise. The fitness professional can perform the talk test with their client throughout the assessment by easily asking their client questions and beginning a conversation. The participant should be working at an intensity that allows them to carry on a conversation without running out of breath. If the individual is unable to do so, this should be recorded and intensity should be decreased.

- Advantages: requires no tools, can be done with most clients regardless of physical and cognitive abilities.
- Disadvantages: If an individual is extremely sedentary he/she may run out of breath well before desired results are achieved. This tool may also require further adaptations for non-verbal participants.

Musculoskeletal Testing

Musculoskeletal testing protocol includes both muscular endurance and muscular strength testing. Adaptations and modifications may be required when using normative protocols. A variety of different tests are also available to use and can be used for all ability levels and ages. It is important to note, that during musculoskeletal testing, the fitness professional must be aware and keep in mind any spine, back or neck ailments that could be contraindicated with the testing provided. Table 4 identifies muscular strength tests available, along with adaptations and recommendations for a variety of abilities. Many of the tests identified in Table 4 follow normative testing protocol. Medicine ball throw is an option to test upper body power similar to the way vertical jump assesses lower body power. This protocol requires the individual to explosively throw the medicine ball as far as possible in a forward direction. See Figure 3 as an example of an individual performing this task.

Table 4. Muscular strength testing

Muscular Strength	Tests Available/ Description	Equipment Options	Adaptations & Recommendations
Grip Strength	Grip Strength Test	Hand Dynamometer	Seated or Standing, can use tensor bandage to assist with maintaining proper grip
Medicine Ball Throw	Record best distance of two trials for test-retest purposes	Measuring tape, medicine ball, masking tape, assistant	Can be performed seated or standing. Vary medicine ball weight depending on client strength. Always retest with same weight
1 RM	1 RM test protocol	Free weights, Velcro Weights, Machine	Warm up set necessary to evaluate technique and determine weight, may not be suitable for participants unable to maintain proper technique or experience fatigue after warm up
8 RM	8 RM test protocol	Free weights, Velcro Weights, Machine	

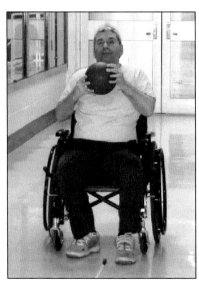

**Figure 3.
Medicine ball throw
assessing upper body
power.**

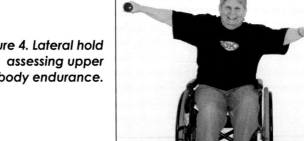

Figure 4. Lateral hold assessing upper body endurance.

Table 5 identifies muscular endurance tests available, along with adaptations and recommendations for a variety of abilities. Several normative tests are available; however the fitness professional may find it useful to perform criterion referenced protocol when assessing muscular endurance on upper and lower body. An example of upper body endurance testing is the lateral hold. Participant holds weight forming a 90 degree angle (if possible) between arm and body for a maximum amount of time. The fitness professional should be looking for upright posture and maintenance of form. See Figure 4 for an example of the lateral hold. For individuals unable to perform lower body endurance testing such as the wall sit (Figure 5), the leg press is a suitable option.

Table 5. Muscular endurance testing

Muscular Endurance	Tests Available	Equipment Options	Adaptations & Recommendations
Upper Body	Push-up test	Mat or raised platform, counter	Can use varied pivot points depending on client (toes, knees, hips)
	Curl-up test	Mat or raised platform, stop watch, metronom	If unable to follow metronome, visual metronome can be used, or allow participant to complete maximum number of curl-ups at own pace. If unable transfer onto mat, rope crunches in chair can be performed following similar protocol
	Seniors curl test	Free weights, Velcro weights	Test developed for older adults, but can be used for persons with mobility impairments. Weights can be modified if needed
	Lateral hold	Free weights or velcro weights, stop watch	Starting position can be varied depending on participant shoulder range of motion – test terminated when unable to maintain starting position
Lower Body	Seniors chair stand test	Standard chair, wheelchair, stop watch	Must be able to stand without pushing off chair or mobility aid
	Leg press	Leg press, stopwatch, counter	Can hold feet in with magnetic plates if needed, tubing or ball can assist in keeping knees aligned with hips
	Wall sit	Stopwatch, wall	Starting position based on balance and strength of participant. Angle of knee can vary between 45° to 90°

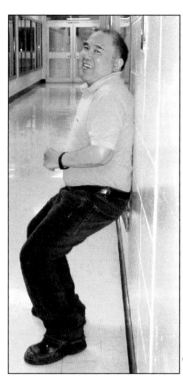

Figure 5.
Wall sit assessing lower
body endurance.

Flexibility and Range of Motion Testing

Flexibility and range of motion (ROM) testing can be performed on clients of all abilities with very little adaptations. Testing should be done on functional muscles only and are commonly used to test shoulder flexion and extension, hamstrings, and the trunk. See Table 6 for a list of tests available, along with adaptations and recommendations for a variety of abilities. Testing trunk control can enhance the fitness professional's knowledge of clients balance and stability within an exercise environment. Please see Figure 6 for an example of lateral trunk flexion.

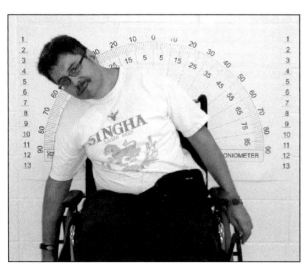

Figure 6.
Wall goniometer
assessing lateral
trunk flexion.

Table 6. Flexibility and range of motion testing

Flexibility & ROM	Tests Available	Equipment Options	Adaptations & Recommendations
Sit and Reach	Sit and reach	Flexometer	Performing tests on individuals with above knee amputations or lower limb paralysis can produce invalid results due to limited function of the hamstrings. If client has asymmetrical upper body functioning, one arm can be used.
Shoulder flexion and extension	Shoulder flexion and extension test	Leighton Flexometer or Goniometer	Passive range of motion or additional assessor guidance may be required.
Trunk	Lateral and forward trunk flexion	Wall goniometer	Can be performed in seated or standing position

Balance testing

Balance should be tested on all individuals who are ambulatory or able to stand independently or using a mobility aid. Understanding an individual's base level of balance will assist in developing a safe and effective program for their needs and abilities. See Table 7 for a list of tests available, along with adaptations and recommendations for a variety of ability levels.

Table 7. Balance testing

Balance	Tests Available	Equipment Options	Adaptations & Recommendations
Functional Balance Assessment	Timed Up and Go	Chair, measuring tape, stop watch	Suitable for participants able to stand up and walk independently or with a mobility aid
	Berg Balance Scale	Chair, measuring tape, step, stopwatch, 15 foot walkway	Only portions of test may be able to be performed depending on ability levels
	Tinetti Performance Orientation Assessment of Balance	Chair, measuring tape, stopwatch	

Interpretation of Results

As mentioned earlier in this chapter, once a test is adapted and modified, it is no longer appropriate to use normative results provided for each test. The majority of tests available for persons with impairments will be able to be used for criterion referenced or test – retest purposes only. For example, results can be used to assist in developing a fitness program that will best meet the individual's current fitness level, goals and abilities.

Re-testing is an effective way to see if your participant has made any improvements and achieved goals. Evaluating progress provides evidence to determine if the program has been successful. It is very important to remember that when re-testing, the fitness professional must replicate the initial test as close as possible to ensure the most accurate results are obtained. Daily variances such as fatigue, mood, motivation, temperature, environment and medications can alter results from test to test.

Summary

All people have the right to be active and live healthier lives. A proper assessment yielding accurate results is the first step to ensuring that each person, no matter their ability, can be active safely and efficiently. By focusing on ones abilities rather than their disability, assessments can be easily modified to ensure that the needs and goals of the participant are met. It is important that fitness professionals have alternate action plans as well as recommended adaptations for cardiovascular, musculoskeletal, anthropometric and balance testing procedures. This ensures the completion of thorough testing and allows for accurate results to be obtained and used for further program development or testing.

References

1. Horvat M., Block M. E., & Kelly L. E. (2007). Developmental and adapted physical activity assessment. Champaign, IL: Human Kinetics

2. Canadian Society of Exercise Physiology (2002). Inclusive fitness & lifestyle services for all disAbilities. Ottawa, ON: Canadian Society of Exercise Physiology.

3. American College of Sports Medicine (2010). ACSM's Resource manual for guidelines for exercise testing and prescription (6th ed.). Baltimore, MD: Lippincott Williams & Wilkins.

4. Rick Hansen Centre (1993). Fitness assessment manual (3rd ed.). Edmonton, AB: Rick Hansen Centre.

5. Canadian Society of Exercise Physiology (2004). The Canadian physical activity, fitness & lifestyle approach (3rd ed.). Ottawa, ON: Canadian Society of Exercise Physiology.

6. Durstine L. J. & Moore G. E. (2003). ACSM's Exercise management for persons with chronic diseases and disabilities (2nd ed.). Champaign, IL: Human Kinetics.

7. Steadward, R. (1998). Musculoskeletal and neurological disabilities: Implications for fitness appraisal, programming and counseling. Canadian Journal of Applied Physiology, 23, 131-165.

Section IV

Exercise Prescription and Programming

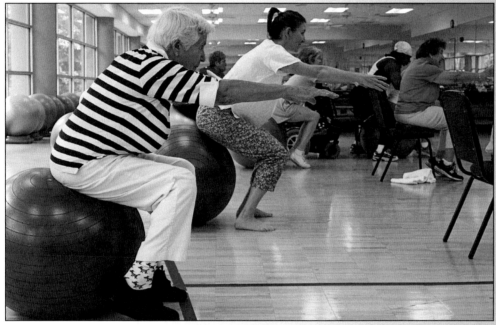

By Carol Kutik, M.A., and Laurie A. Malone, Ph.D.

Carol Kutik has an M.A. in Exercise Physiology from the University of Alabama at Birmingham. Her certifications include: Personal Trainer and AHFS (Advanced Health and Fitness Specialist) from The American Council on Exercise, as well as CIFT (Certified Inclusive Fitness Trainer) from the American College of Sports Medicine. As Director of Fitness and Health Promotion for Lakeshore Foundation, Carol is responsible for oversight and development of fitness and personal training programs, as well as creating and implementing health promotion activities related to nutrition, exercise, and health education.

Laurie A. Malone, Ph.D., has served as Director of Research and Education at Lakeshore Foundation since 2002. Her research utilizes a multi-disciplinary approach to examine the impact of physical activity on the lives of persons with disability. With Lakeshore Foundation's designation as a U.S. Olympic and Paralympic Training Site, Dr. Malone is responsible for providing sport science services to National team athletes. She serves as a Health Promotion Research Specialist for the National Center on Health, Physical Activity, and Disability, on the Board of Directors for the International Federation for Adapted Physical Activity, and founding member of International Network for the Advancement of Paralympic Sport through Science.

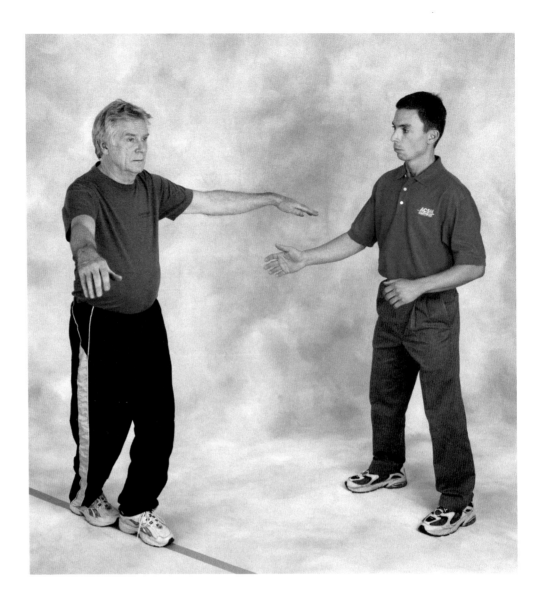

Section Overview

This section provides the Certified Inclusive Fitness Trainer (CIFT) with the key elements needed to develop and implement a safe and effective, individualized exercise program for persons with a physical, sensory, or cognitive disability. Guidelines for developing an exercise program defined by the mode, intensity, duration, frequency and progression of training are discussed. Principles of specificity, overload, progression, consistency, goal setting and principles of adaptation are reviewed. Additionally, this section presents relevant and specific guidelines for modifying basic principles of conditioning for the development of exercise programs for persons with disabilities to enable them to engage in healthy, active lifestyles.

Recommending exercise programs for persons with disabilities should always begin with an initial consultation and assessment, as explained in Section 3. It is imperative that the client be an active partner in setting goals and developing a program that helps to meet those goals. Some clients may be interested in improving mobility and independence, or be better able to carry out daily activities independently, while others may wish to improve performance in a specific task or recreational activity. The exercise program should be an ongoing process which continues to assess and modify the client's response to the training program. This is particularly important with individuals who have progressive disorders or who may experience a decline in function. Of utmost importance to the CIFT is to understand that while general guidelines may be offered for certain impairment types, each individual may respond to training differently. The CIFT should always be able to recognize pertinent precautions and contraindications, but never predetermine exercise programming prior to consultation and assessment of the client.

This section briefly addresses cardiovascular, resistance, flexibility, balance and stability training. It addresses the basic components of a training session and begins the process of program design in terms of session components and exercise selection. Functional exercises for each component will be provided.

The CIFT should be able to identify the anatomical structures of the musculoskeletal system that are affected by a client's disability and design a training program that addresses specific behaviors as well as functional abilities and limitations to ensure the success of the program.

Overload and Progression

A training program will produce limited results when a client does not experience overload regularly. Overload requires that the structural and functional adaptation of a system of the body be stressed beyond the level to which it is accustomed and is generally defined by four variables: (1) frequency, or how often the exercise is performed; (2) intensity, or how hard the exercise is; (3) duration, or how long an exercise is performed; and (4) mode, or what type of exercise is performed.

Progression is defined as an increase in workload in order to achieve continual improvements in fitness. Strength and endurance gains in resistance training should progressively overload the muscular system by manipulating the following variables:
- increasing the intensity or weight (resistance)
- increasing the number of repetitions or sets
- decreasing the rest period between sets
- adding exercises for individual muscle groups

Appropriate strength training loads are determined by the client's fitness level, goals, and functional ability. The one repetition maximum (1RM) testing method is defined as the maximum weight that can be lifted in a single effort. While this method yields a precise and objective assessment of strength, it is contraindicated for most individuals in a general fitness program because it imposes a high risk of injury. However, for healthy active individuals such as Paralympic athletes, 1RM testing under the supervision of an experienced trainer may be appropriate. For those in a general fitness program, it is safer to predict 1RM by performing a submaximal set of repetitions (4-10 reps). For beginners, low training loads are recommended to strengthen the tendons and ligaments for increased loads later in training. Certain individuals with progressive conditions, joint instability (*e.g.*, Down syndrome), pain with movement (*e.g.*, arthritis), or a likelihood of developing disabling fatigue (*e.g.*, multiple sclerosis) should avoid strength training to exhaustion. The CIFT should closely monitor client discomfort with such conditions, individualizing the rate of progression. More frequent, shorter sessions may be appropriate for those with extreme fatigue or weakness. Limits to strength training gains will be strongly influenced by the stage and nature of the condition.

Specificity

In order to reach a specific goal or produce a specific result, the client has to follow a specific type of training. Increases in aerobic capacity are related to the volume of muscle utilized in stressing the cardiovascular system. Increases in strength and muscle endurance must stress the metabolic pathways (aerobic and anaerobic) and involve a specific muscle group and muscle fiber recruitment. Improvements in balance are achieved by stressing the somatosensory, visual, and vestibular systems.

Consistency

Loss of training benefits, or detraining, will occur when exercise is discontinued, because training effects are transient and reversible. Certain persons with disabilities (neuromuscular impairments), which have periods of exacerbation and remission, will likely experience intermittent detraining. The CIFT should play a role in coaching clients to cope with the frustration caused by interruptions. The trainer can help clients develop realistic goals and help maintain a focus on the importance of a healthy lifestyle (*e.g.,* physical activity, proper nutrition, smoking cessation, stress management, adequate rest).

Goal Setting

After the initial consultation and assessment, the most valuable tool the CIFT has is goal setting which is the first essential step in developing an exercise program. This should be a joint effort and is when the client-trainer rapport is best established. While some conditions associated with a disability may limit progress, the fitness professional can help the client establish realistic goals by maintaining emphasis on abilities and avoiding focus on limitations.

Goals are best met by defining short term and long term desires and by using the S.M.A.R.T. method. S.M.A.R.T. goals are Specific, Measureable, Attainable, Relevant, and Time-Bound. After the client sets goals, help him or her understand the factors that influence their ability to achieve their goals. Regular documentation will keep goals on track and can serve as a motivational tool for the client as they experience progress toward meeting specific goals. Also, the documentation is valuable information to share with the client's healthcare provider.

Adaptation

While specific adaptations and modifications may be relevant for a particular client, many people with disabilities lead independent lives and require very few accommodations. Adapt only when necessary, and adapt on an individual basis. The use of a wheelchair, prosthetic device, cane, walker, and/or service animal may be of assistance. In addition, specialized grips, straps, leg supports or wheelchair accessible fitness equipment provide a range of opportunities. The CIFT should research the possibilities for their particular client and stay abreast of new developments. Adaptations may be temporary until the person can learn skills to participate in a standard or typical way. Adaptations should make sense. Ask yourself at the end of the day, "Is the program safe, is the client satisfied, and is the client experiencing success?"

Common Terms Associated with Disability

This section will review some of the characteristics of various disabilities that may alter exercise response. It is important for the CIFT to understand alterations to biomechanics and kinesiology, as well as changes to anatomy and basic physiology of body systems that may result from various disabilities and health conditions. It also includes exercise considerations specific to various disabilities and health conditions.

Each group of disabilities may have a distinct exercise response, such as neuromuscular conditions alter messages to and from the brain, musculoskeletal conditions affect joint and muscle properties, and cognitive conditions may affect the ability to remember program components. These responses may not be mutually exclusive. Exercise programming will, in turn, be affected by such responses. Daily fluctuations in responses should be monitored.

References

1. Durstine, J. Larry, Moore, Geoffery E., Painter, Patricia, L., & Roberts, Scott O. (Eds.). (2009). ACSM's Exercise Management for Persons with Chronic Diseases and Disabilities (3rd ed.). Champaign, IL: Human Kinetics. Miller, Patricia D., (Ed.). (1995). Fitness Programming and Physical Disability. Champaign, IL: Human Kinetics.

2. National Center on Physical Activity & Disability. (n.d.). Are You at Risk? Understanding BMI and What it Means to You. Retrieved January 06, 2012, from http://www.ncpad.org/fact_sheet.php?sheet=394

3. National Center on Health, Physical Activity and Disability. (n.d.). Common Overuse Injuries in Wheelchair Users. Retrieved January 6, 2012, from http://www.ncpad.org/exercise/fact_sheet.php?sheet=109

4. National Center on Health, Physical Activity and Disability. (n.d.). Person-First Language and Disability Awareness: Interaction Tips for the Fitness Professional. Retrieved January 06, 2012, from http://www.ncpad.org/exercise/fact_sheet.php?sheet=680

5. National Center on Health, Physical Activity and Disability (n.d.). Resistance Training for Persons with Physical Disabilities. Retrieved January 06, 2012, from http://www.ncpad.org/exercise/fact_sheet.php?sheet=107

6. National Center on Health, Physical Activity and Disability. (n.d.). Use of the International Classification of Functioning, Disability and Health (ICF) to Prepare Individualized Exercise Prescriptions for People with Disabilities. Retrieved January 06, 2012, from http://www.ncpad.org/fitt/fact_sheet.php?sheet=459

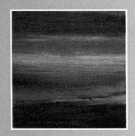

CHAPTER 12

General Exercise Program Design Considerations

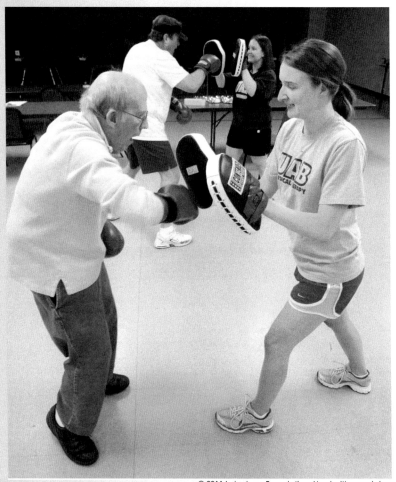

According to the *2008 Physical Activity Guidelines for Individuals with Disabilities*, people with disabilities tend to live more sedentary lifestyles and have been found to be at much greater risk of developing chronic diseases and secondary conditions associated with inactive lifestyles. Secondary conditions can be directly or indirectly associated with the primary disability. However, in many cases, they are preventable with regular physical activity and an overall healthy lifestyle.

Adults with disabilities, who are able to, should perform the following:

- Aerobic activity for ≥ 150 minutes/week (moderate intensity) or 75 minutes (vigorous intensity) or equivalent combination, performed in episodes of ≥ 10 minutes and spread throughout the week
- Muscle-strengthening activities of moderate or high intensity that involve all major muscle groups on ≥ 2 days/week

When adults with disabilities are not able to meet the physical activity guidelines, they should engage in regular physical activity according to abilities and avoid inactivity. In addition, they should consult their healthcare provider about amounts and types of physical activity that are appropriate for their abilities. Most importantly, providing education and activity options that will motivate and increase exercise adherence is critical in the role as a CIFT.

Based on the basic principles of conditioning and training, utilize these guidelines when developing an exercise program for a person with a disability:

- Obtain medical clearance if deemed necessary (see Section 3)
- Assess a baseline to establish an appropriate beginning intensity and identify strong/weak muscle systems. Know the potential side effects of medications on exercise
- Consider overload, progression, specificity, goal setting and documentation, and relevant adaptations to customize the program to meet the client's needs and abilities
- Work with the client to establish S.M.A.R.T. goals and keep meticulous records
- Establish a wellness program for overall health that addresses all of the components of fitness: cardiovascular, strength, flexibility, balance, posture, muscular imbalance, body composition, coordination, and physical function

Basic Safety Considerations

Some basic safety considerations hold true for all clients. Exercise should stop if any of the following are present:

- Pain
- Discomfort
- Nausea
- Dizziness
- Chest pain
- Lightheadedness
- Irregular heart rate
- Shortness of breath
- Clammy hands

Plenty of fluids (especially water) should be encouraged and appropriate clothing is essential. There are additional safety considerations that should be addressed with a client with a disability:

- Pressure sores – may require medical attention and the client should not exercise.
- Increased or unusual spasticity may require alteration of exercise setup, technique, or training protocol.
- Encourage client to empty bowel or bladder before starting exercise (including leg bags).
- Watch areas with poor sensation for signs of redness and swelling. Bones of weak limbs can be at a high risk of breaking with less force than normal.
- Wheelchair users should be able to transfer independently and safely to accessible equipment. Anyone providing assistance with transfer should be trained in safe transfer.
- Thermoregulation, the ability to maintain body temperature may be compromised, especially in individuals with multiple sclerosis (MS) or spinal cord injury (SCI). Monitor environmental temperature, wear appropriate clothing, drink plenty of fluids, and make use of fans or water spray.
- Autonomic dysreflexia, a sudden rise in blood pressure, is a risk for persons with SCI of T6 or above. Symptoms include profuse sweating, sudden elevation of blood pressure, shivering, headache, bradycardia, and nausea. If symptoms of autonomic dysreflexia are present, stop exercise immediately, and encourage the client to check for problems with catheter or pressure sore and seek medical attention if symptoms continue. Monitoring BP and having the client empty bladder/catheter prior to exercise may prevent this condition.
- Orthostatic hypotension, a drop in blood pressure when maintaining an upright position may occur in persons with SCI as well as other cardiovascular conditions. Signs are dizziness, nausea, and light headedness. If orthostatic hypotension occurs, the client should lie in a supine position with feet elevated. Preventive measures include the avoidance of quick movements, especially upright ones, maintaining proper hydration, and the use of compression stockings or abdominal binder.

- Incontinence is a concern for many persons with disabilities and chronic health conditions and should be addressed appropriately.
- Transfer ability is key in determining the exercise program for any client using a wheelchair or assistive device. Independent transfer should be highly encouraged and taught. It may not be within the scope of practice of the CIFT to transfer clients. Transfer assistance should be only be performed by an individual trained in safe transfer technique. Use of transfer tools (*e.g.,* sliding boards) can allow for the individual to transfer independently or to make it easier for the attendant.
- The role of aids must be explicit, the client is in control of the type of assistance provided and training of the attendant is a joint responsibility of client and fitness center staff.

Specific Considerations

Wheelchair Users

The repetitive motions associated with wheelchair usage are a risk for developing overuse injuries and muscular imbalance. Rotator cuff and shoulder impingement are of particular concern, as are carpal tunnel syndrome and lateral epicondylitis. Poor trunk musculature can exacerbate imbalance and increase the risk of falling from the chair during exercise or everyday activity. Chest pressing exercises will strengthen the muscles used for wheeling and transfer, and pulling exercises, such as rowing and lat pulls will improve seated posture and imbalance between anterior and posterior muscle groups. Practical exercises including internal and external rotation, shoulder abduction and extension, and seated push-ups can prevent pressure sores and increase transfer ability. Wheelchair users should know how to transfer safely to accessible equipment; this requires training of the biceps and triceps. Use of transfers throughout an exercise routine (on and off machines) is important to consider and should be factored into the number and type of exercises performed.

Individuals with Spinal Cord Injury

Complete or incomplete impairment of the spinal cord will result in loss of sensation and motor function at the point of injury and below. In an incomplete injury, there is some function below the injury site, while in a complete injury there is no function below the injury site. Autonomic dysreflexia, spasticity, orthostatic hypotension, thermoregulation, incontinence, pressure ulcers or skin breakdown and heart rate response are of particular concern in working with a person with SCI.

Since the level of injury determines functional ability, the need for and utilization of adaptive equipment will vary. Velcro straps, gloves, elastic bands, and/or tubing will allow the use of resistance and cardiovascular equipment by persons within a large range of functional ability. Depending on the level of injury, trunk balance may be compromised; core strengthening exercises targeting remaining muscle mass are essential. Strength training exercises should be performed as close to full range of movement as possible; assistance may be needed in securing grips and to achieve full ROM. The ultimate goal, however, should be independence in exercise performance.

Frequent position changes are essential in limiting pressure sores and skin breakdown. It is wise to communicate regularly with the client in order to check for such breakdowns because the lack of sensation makes the presence of these conditions unrecognizable. In this regard client education is important so they know what to look for and understand the potential 'risks' of exercise. Proactive measures such as advising on clothing, etc., can be beneficial to prevent skin irritations. Additionally, seated push-ups are recommended to release pressure and skin irritation.

Since ADL's may require regular recruitment of muscle groups required to move through ADL activity, the program should focus on activities that use different muscle groups. Shoulder, wrist, hip and chest tightness are common; these muscle groups should be stretched, while antagonistic muscle groups strengthened.

Nash et al. provide guidelines for exercise prescription and monitoring of exercise intensity in persons with SCI.[6] SCI can impact both maximum and training heart rate. Persons with tetraplegia (quadriplegia) often do not achieve age predicted maximum heart rate; typical maximum heart rate (MHR) falls within a range of 115-130. Persons with paraplegia with injury T1 to T6 may also have a blunted MHR response and a non-linear relationship between exercise HR and VO_2. Therefore using HR max or HRR (heart rate reserve) as methods for fitness assessment or intensity estimation are less valid. If available, an arm exercise test will measure peak VO_2 and provide a more accurate MHR. A prescription can then be derived to target workloads at the desired percentage of max. RPE is a viable option for establishing the intensity component of the prescription.[2]

For injuries at or below T2, eliciting a MHR response closer to age-predicted is likely, as HR response is closely linear with VO_2. Exercise prescriptions can be computed using HRR, HR max, VO_2, or RPE. Another option for intensity estimation involves use of the CDC recommended talk test, which although not validated in persons with SCI, still offers a simple, easy-to-use estimate of exercise intensity.[4]

Both the HRR and HR max methods require an estimated or measured HR max. HR max is estimated by subtracting the person's age in years from 220 (220 - age).[1] Table 1 defines the moderate and vigorous intensity RPE and HR ranges for ages 20 - 80 years based on the age-estimated HR max. HRR requires a resting HR (HR rest) measure; ideally, taken immediately upon awakening in the morning. The equation to establish upper and lower limits of the target range for the HRR method is as follows: upper/lower limit = HR max + (intensity * HRR), where HRR = HR max − HR rest. Intensity is entered as a percentage of HR max (*i.e.*, 70% = 0.70). Two different intensities are used to define the upper and lower limits of the desired target range. A full description and explanation of the available methods can be found in Chapter 7 in the *ACSM Guidelines for Exercise Testing and Prescription*.[1, 6]

Spina Bifida

Spina bifida results from an abnormality in neural tube development inutero. Weakness can occur in areas that have damaged nerve control. Compromised areas are typically in the muscles to the abdomen, legs, bowel and bladder. Additional considerations are posture, latex allergies, incontinence, thermoregulation, pressure sores, presence of a shunt

Table 1. Target heart rate ranges for moderate and vigorous activity based on estimated peak heart rate for persons with injuries at T2 and below. RPE targets are applicable for all persons.[6]

Age (yrs)	Moderate activity (bpm)	Vigorous activity (bpm)
	PE = 12 - 13	RPE = 14 - 16
20	110–140	140–160
25	107–137	137–156
30	105–133	133–152
35	102–130	130–148
40	99–126	126–144
45	96–123	123–140
50	94–119	119–136
55	91–116	116–132
60	88–112	112–128
65	85–109	109–124
70	83–105	105–120
75	80–102	102–116
80	77–98	98–112

Note: bpm = beats per minute. RPE intensity is based on Borg's 6-20 scale.

to divert excess cerebrospinal fluid from the head (hydrocephalus), and fractures in weak limbs as a result of osteoporosis. If a shunt is present, the client should discuss exercise activity with their doctor, and care must be taken to avoid trauma to the shunt and tubing during exercise. Spasticity may occur below the site of injury and can be aggravated by cold air, urinary tract infection, and physical exercise. Functional muscle mass and movement encompasses a wide range, so will the exercise program. Exercise can prevent deconditioning, promote function and endurance, help prevent obesity, decrease constipation, improve infection resistance, and improve mood, while reducing stress, and helping to prevent diabetes and heart disease. Common areas of tightness for the client with spina bifida are hamstrings, adductors, hip flexors, foot flexors and back extensors.

Amputation

Amputation is typically classified as above the knee, below the knee, above the elbow, or below the elbow. The level of amputation determines functional ability, yet with a well-fitted prosthesis, most individuals with amputation can utilize traditional exercise equipment. Standing cardiovascular activities may be difficult at first as balance and stabilization may have been compromised; therefore, utilization of adaptive equipment may be appropriate until the client becomes better accustomed to changes and remaining muscle groups experience neuromuscular and physiological improvements in function. The client should give proper care to the amputation site, checking regularly for pressure sores and skin breakdown; equipment chosen should not aggravate the site. Remaining muscle mass will have an affect on muscle group recruitment and may require greater energy expenditure for cardiovascular and resistance exercise.

The exercise program should include all of the basic conditioning components: cardio, strength, flexibility, balance and agility. Individuals with lower limb amputation may require alternative activities/exercises as it is common that daily prosthetic use may not be possible. They may require use of a wheelchair one day but not another. Progression will be determined by close monitoring of exercise response and feedback by the client.

Cerebral Palsy

Cerebral palsy (CP) is a non-progressive condition that affects muscle control and coordination caused by damage to the brain in utero or shortly after birth (up to age three).

Types and degrees of CP are classified as:
- Spastic: (70% to 80% of cases) accompanied by a high degree of muscle tone
- Athetoid: (10% to 20%) accompanied by uncontrolled flailing movements
- Ataxia: (10%) accompanied by balance and coordination impairments
- Mixed may be a combination of types

Functional ability and muscle mass recruitment is highly individualized; functional assessment is imperative in developing the exercise program.[6] Special considerations include spasticity, pain and fatigue, movement alterations, challenged balance and coordination, involuntary movements, seizures, incontinence, scoliosis, and problems with speech, vision, hearing, reflex development and cognition.[8] In the presence of a shunt to divert excess cerebrospinal fluid from the head (hydrocephalus), the client should discuss exercise activity with their doctor and care must be taken to avoid trauma to the shunt and tubing during exercise. A higher than average incidence of osteoporosis is common in persons with CP, therefore, the exercise program should incorporate modes which minimize risk of bone injury.

Common areas of tightness include the hip, shoulder adductors, and plantar flexors. All muscle groups (including spastic) should be strengthened, with a focus on the weak (hemiplegic) side. The goal of training should be to restore muscle balance. Opposing muscle groups should be worked in the same exercise session. A "push-pull" routine, such as the bench press, or other chest press motion, followed by rowing is one example of targeting opposing muscle groups. Spasticity in a muscle group may habitually place the limb in a position that shortens the muscle on one side of the joint and lengthens it on the opposing side. Note that spasticity may also be present in head injury, stroke and incomplete spinal injury. If contractures are present, movement should be limited to within the capability of the client and avoidance of overstretching contractures is important as it poses a risk of injury.

In persons with cerebral palsy and other related conditions, it is important to not confuse speech impairment with cognitive impairment or intelligence. However, keep in mind that documented cognitive impairment may affect functional ability and require a differ-ent form of communication.

Brain Injury

Whether due to a closed head (stroke, concussion) or open head (bullet, wound) trauma, brain injury can range from mild to severe. Considerations may include headaches, photo sensitivity, sleep disturbances, impaired speech, fatigue, and seizures. Paresis, paralysis or spasticity will challenge movement, and behavioral and emotional issues may be accompanied by mood swings, depression, anxiety and apathy. Vision and hearing may be affected, as well as balance and agility. Overall coordination issues may be present depending on which areas of the brain were damaged. Adherence to the pre-scribed exercise routine and fitness center etiquette should be monitored.

Stroke

Also called cardiovascular accident (CVA) or "brain attack," a stroke results from a sudden disruption of blood supply to the brain by blood clot or hemorrhage. The degree of affect on function is determined by the location and severity of the disruption. As with all disabilities, functional ability is individualized, necessitating a comprehensive assess-ment and history prior to exercise programming. Stroke is a non-progressive condition hence, barring the development of secondary conditions, total recovery is attainable by some while others may experience little progression. The major goal of conditioning for the person that has had a stroke is to regain as much function as possible and to gain or maintain independence, while discouraging risk factors for a second stroke.

Hypertension is often present in the client that has experienced a stroke. Blood pressure should be stable before beginning an exercise program, and it is important for blood pres-sure to be under control and monitored regularly. ACSM dictates that exercise be stopped if BP reaches 220/110. The CIFT should monitor BP before, during and after exercise and be aware of orthostatic hypotension that may develop. Intensity of cardiovascular exercise is most appropriately measured by using RPE or the Rate Pressure Product (RPP). The product should be under 200, using the following equation:

$$RPP = Systolic\ BP\ x\ HR/100$$

Hemiparesis or hemiplegic (when one side is involved) is a major consideration in choosing exercise modalities. Training should strengthen the affected side, as well as main-tain strength in the non-affected side. A mitt, splint or assistive grip (velcro straps for hands/feet) will allow the affected side to move through the ROM. A good starting point is 70% of 10 RM for 1 set of 15-20 reps. If 25 reps can be performed in 2 consecutive sets, increase the weight by 10%. Since hypertension may be present, always avoid the Valsalva maneuver and keep intensity in the low to moderate range. A NuStep® is an ex-cellent choice for cardiovascular training, since its synchronous movement of upper and lower body allows the affected side to be passively moved through the range of motion, propelled by the non-affected side. Hemiparesis or hemiplegia may result in poor trunk and postural balance and stability, therefore balance training should be an integral component of the exercise program.

Multiple Sclerosis

Multiple sclerosis is an autoimmune disease that affects the Central Nervous System (CNS). The myelin sheath of the nerves is damaged or destroyed, which affects the function of the brain, spinal cord and optic nerve. It is most common in individuals between the ages of 20 to 50 years.

MS is categorized by the following:
- *Relapsing Remitting*: the most common form, characterized by exacerbations of symptoms, followed by periods of partial or complete recovery
- *Primary Progressive*: progressive with continuous worsening of symptoms
- *Secondary Progressive*: begins with relapsing remitting and steadily worsens; may or may not have exacerbations and remissions
- *Progressive Relapsing*: Steadily worsens from initial onset with or without remission

Common symptoms and responses include a blunted HR and reduced BP, an abnormal sensation of numbness, tingling, and pain which can be symmetrical or asymmetrical, and excess fatigue. Additionally, movement is impaired by tight muscle groups (*e.g.,* hip flexors, hamstrings, calves, trunk and chest), difficulty ambulating, muscle weakness and challenged balance and coordination, increasing the risk of falls. In some cases, with progression of the disease individuals may become dependent on the use of a power wheelchair. Vision, including painful eye movement, blurring or loss of vision may also be present. Of particular concern in exercise programming is decreased heat tolerance.[11] The CIFT should minimize exposure to high temperatures, including land and aquatic exercise. Aquatic exercise should be conducted in a pool with a temperature of less than 84 degrees. A "cool vest" can provide significant relief from increased body temperatures. Exercise should be performed in the coolest environment possible with the presence of air conditioning and fans.

The exercise program must monitor the client continually for fatigue and proper hydration. Free weight exercises can pose added risk when sensory deficits are present. Appropriate gloves and straps enhance safe gripping. Because of the risk of falling in clients experiencing balance and coordination challenges, static and dynamic balance training should be included in the program.

Muscular Dystrophy

Muscular dystrophy is a hereditary progressive degeneration of skeletal and/or involuntary muscle, which leads to a progressive loss of strength and decreased function.[9]

Diminished cardiac function will decrease oxygen delivery during exercise, so cardiovascular exercise should not be strenuous, but rather, focus on duration. A stress echocardiogram and electrocardiogram are recommended prior to beginning exercise. RPE is recommended for monitoring intensity during exercise with 12-14 on the Borg scale as a target zone. Good choices are short walking sessions, stationary cycling, arm ergometry and swimming.

Spasticity and contractures must be addressed, as well as attention to tight hip flexors, hamstrings, calves and chest muscles. Muscle weakness typically begins in the lower extremities and moves upward, all affecting balance and coordination and increasing the risk of falls. Resistance training should focus on multi-joint activity to improve function, and resistance should be light; increase reps vs. intensity. Increase reps vs. intensity and avoid overload.

Active or passive ROM exercises are appropriate. However, overstretching should be avoided. Static stretches for tightness and contracture can be performed several times/day and should be slow, controlled and held for 10-20 seconds.

Intellectual Disability (ID)

Understanding levels of cognition and the possible presence of heart conditions are of utmost importance to the CIFT. Low IQ (< 70) and adaptive behavior will affect memory, learning, and processing of information. Allow extra time to complete a task, and present specific activities, in an easily understood format that include only one or two steps. Use of alternate/varied communication strategies may be needed. A reward system will reinforce small accomplishments and develop a feeling of success and accomplishment in the client.

Increasing cardiovascular fitness can be challenging, especially in persons with heart conditions. The ultimate goal is to exercise at moderate and vigorous intensities, so that improvements can be achieved. Start slowly and begin with smaller, more frequent sessions, and then progress to moderate sessions of 30 minutes and vigorous sessions of 20 minutes. Choose activities that are easy to learn, such as walking or stationary cycling, but don't avoid more challenging activities (*e.g.,* dancing, swimming) if the client demonstrates a desire and ability to learn and perform the activities safely. Some persons with ID may experience MHR less 8 to 20% lower than predicted, making subjective monitoring, such as RPE or the Talk Test more appropriate.

Muscular strength and endurance are essential for carrying out ADL's and the type of resistance program selected should include overload and progression that the client can perform. *Atlantoaxial instability*, a loose ligament between C1 and C2, is present in up to 17% of individuals with Down syndrome, and can lead to slippage of cervical alignment and spinal injury. Exercise training can increase muscle strength and agility in persons with Down Syndrome, however, certain activities should be avoided including diving, heading a soccer ball, etc.[7] Hypermobility can cause joints to stretch past the normal ROM so flexibility exercises are not recommended. Flexibility training is also contraindicated for individuals with hypotonia, as it can further loosen joints and cause injury.

Autism

Autism is a developmental disorder, with impairments ranging from mild to severe. Social interaction and communication along with the presence of atypical behaviors frequently known as stimming are common. Cognitive impairment may or may not be present, as well as difficulty in sensory integration. Hypo or hyperactive responses to the five basic senses, as well as the proprioceptive and vestibular systems may exacerbate distractions to stimuli. Eye contact may be avoided and reciprocal communication challenged. The CIFT must possess extraordinary communication skills focusing on verbal to non-verbal, repetitive use of language and maintaining conversations. Use of simple, direct cueing, pictorial systems or written cue cards can be quite effective. Statements such as first XXXX then YYYY are commonly used. Fine and gross motor skills may be impaired, making movement and exercise technique difficult. Nonetheless, the exercise program can encompass all of the major components and principles of fitness, with close and continual monitoring of exercise response, client understanding and feedback, and alignment with goals. Social skills and communication issues are the main concerns. Individuals with autism are often visual learners. Also, individuals with autism may possess low muscle tone and reduced muscular strength. Motor skills may or may not be delayed.

Visual and Hearing Impairments

Visual or hearing impairments do not alter the basic conditioning principles of fitness. They do require an additional assessment to determine the level of impairment. Visual impairment can range from low/limited vision to total blindness. Hearing impairment can range from mild loss to profound deafness.

When working with a client with visual impairment, it is important to allow time for exploration and learning a new environment. Always identify yourself and others when the level of impairment prevents recognition, speak in a normal tone, indicate when you are moving and give specific directions such as "to the right 10 feet." Assess the physical environment for availability of large, colorful print or braille materials, and use tactile guides for moving from one piece of equipment or area to another. If these aids are not available, investigate the possibility of equipping braille or tactile and visual enhancements to the workout equipment and area. Be familiar with how and where to obtain additional and alternative materials.

Find out how a client with a hearing impairment prefers to communicate, (*e.g.,* hearing aid, reading lips, interpreter, or sign language). Be familiar with sources for communication aids, and don't be hesitant to let the person know if you are having difficulty understanding. Always speak directly to the person and in a normal tone. Balance may be an issue, especially in clients with a large degree of hearing loss. Hearing aids and cochlear implants may be removed for physical activity, which could affect communication.

References

1. American College of Sports Medicine (2010). ACSM's Guidelines For Exercise Testing and Prescription (8th Edition). Philadelphia, PA: Lippincott Williams & Wilkins. 152-180, 241-244.

2. Borg, G. (1982). Psychophysical bases of perceived exertion. Med Sci Sports Exerc, 14, 377-381, 1982.

3. Cooney JK, Law RJ, Matschke V, Lemmey AB, Moore JP, Ahmad Y, Jones JG, Maddison P, Thom JM. Benefits of exercise in rheumatoid arthritis. J Aging Res. 2011 Feb 13;2011:681640.

4. Durstine, J. Larry, Moore, Geoffery E., Painter, Patricia, L., & Roberts, Scott O. (Eds.). (2009). ACSM's Exercise Management for Persons with Chronic Diseases and Disabilities (3rd ed.). Champaign, IL: Human Kinetics.

5. Foster, C., Porcari, J. P., Anderson, J., Paulson, M., Smaczny, D., Webber, H., Doberstein, S. T., & Udermann, B. (2008). The talk test as a marker of exercise training intensity. J Cardiopulm Rehabil Prev, 28, 24-32.

6. Hombergen SP, Huissstede BM, Streur MF, Stam HJ, Slaman J, Bussmann JB, van den Berg-Emons RJ. Impact of cerebral palsy on health-related physical fitness in adults: systematic review. Arch Phys Med Rehabil. 2012 May;93(5):871-81.

7. Lin HC, Wuang YP. Strength and agility training in adolescents with Down syndrome: A randomized controlled trial. Res Dev Disabil. 2012 Nov;33(6):2236-44. Epub 2012 Jul 21.

8. Malone LA, Vogtle LK. Pain and fatigue consistency in adults with cerebral palsy. Disabil Rehabil. 2010;32(5):385-91.

9. Markert CD, Ambrosio F, Call JA, Grange RW. Exercise and Duchenne muscular dystrophy: toward evidence-based exercise prescription. Muscle Nerve. 2011 Apr;43(4):464-78. doi: 10.1002/mus.21987.

10. Miller, Patricia D., (Eds.). (1995). Fitness Programming and Physical Disability. Champaign, IL: Human Kinetics.

11. Motl RW, Pilutti LA. The benefits of exercise training in multiple sclerosis. Nat Rev Neurol. 2012 Sep 3;8(9):487-97. doi: 10.1038/nrneurol.2012.136. Epub 2012 Jul 24.

12. Nash, M. S., Horton, J. A., Cowan, R. E., & Malone, L. A. (Dec, 2011). Recreational and therapeutic exercise after spinal cord injury. In D. I. Campagnolo, S. Kirshblum, M. S. Nash, R. F. Heary, & P. H. Gorman (Eds.), Spinal Cord Medicine (2nd Edition). Chicago, IL: Lippincott Williams & Wilkins.

13. National Center on Health, Physical Activity and Disability (n.d.). Acquired Brain Injury. Retrieved January 06, 2012, from http://www.ncpad.org/disability/fact_sheet.php?sheet=111.

14. National Center on Health, Physical Activity and Disability (n.d.). Amputation. Retrieved January 06, 2012, from http://www.ncpad.org/disability/fact_sheet.php?sheet=324.

15. National Center on Health, Physical Activity and Disability (n.d.). Autism and Considerations in Recreation and Physical Activity Settings. Retrieved January 06, 2012, from http://www.ncpad.org/disability/fact_sheet.php?sheet=366.

16. National Center on Health, Physical Activity and Disability (n.d.). Cerebral Palsy and Exercise. Retrieved January 06, 2012, from http://www.npcad.org/disability/fact_sheet.php?shseet=119.

17. National Center on Health, Physical Activity and Disability (n.d.). Intellectual Disabilities and Fitness. Retrieved January 06, 2012, from http://www.ncpad.org/disability/fact_sheet.php?sheet=143.

18. National Center on Health, Physical Activity and Disability (n.d.). Multiple sclerosis: Designing an exercise program. Retrieved January 06, 2012, from http://www.npcad.org/disability/fact_sheet.php?sheet=187.

19. National Center on Health, Physical Activity and Disability (n.d.). Resistance Training for Persons with Physical Disabilities. Retrieved January 06, 2012, from http://www.ncpad.org/exercise/fact_sheet.php?sheet=107.

20. National Center on Health, Physical Activity and Disability (n.d.). Spinal Cord Injury and Exercise. Retrieved January 06, 2012, from http://www.ncpad.org/disability/fact_sheet.php?sheet=130.

21. National Center on Health, Physical Activity and Disability (n.d.). Stroke. Retrieved January 06, 2012, from http://www.ncpad.org/disability/fact_sheet.php?sheet=132.

22. National Center on Health, Physical Activity and Disability (n.d.) Muscular Dystrophy. Retrieved January 06, 2012, from http://www.ncpad.org/disability/fact_sheet.php?sheet=73.

23. Rimmer JH, Marques AC. Physical activity for people with disabilities. Lancet. 2012 Jul 21;380(9838):193-5.

24. Rimmer JH, Schiller W, Chen MD. Effects of disability-associated low energy expenditure deconditioning syndrome. Exerc Sport Sci Rev. 2012 Jan;40(1):22-9. doi: 10.1097/JES.0b013e31823b8b82.

25. Thompson, W. R., Bushman, B. A., Desch, J., & Kravitz, L. (Eds.). (2010). ACSM's Resources for the Personal Trainer (3rd ed.). Philadelphia, PA: Lippincott Williams & Wilkins.

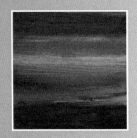

CHAPTER 13

Flexibility and Balance Programs

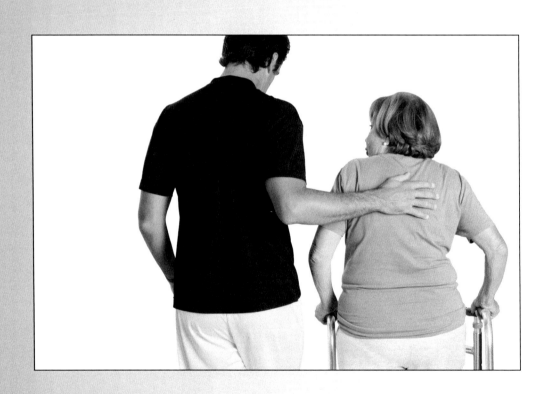

Flexibility

Because of its value in maintaining muscle balance and functional ability, flexibility is a critical component of the exercise program for persons with disabilities. Establishing optimal range of motion (ROM) for specific joints may not be as appropriate as is identifying functional ROM. The goal of flexibility training is to maintain the integrity of the joints and improve the ability to carry out activities of daily living (ADLs). Flexibility training can also prevent joint contracture, pain and injury.

The stretch reflex, or the ability to stretch, is regulated by sensory receptors within skeletal muscle the muscle spindle and the Golgi Tendon Organ (GTO). The muscle spindle is activated in response to changes in muscle length and its activation facilitates a contraction of the muscle when it reaches a certain length. The GTO, located in the tendon, activates when it senses contraction in the muscle and causes the tendon to relax in order to prevent injury. Disabilities involving impairment to motor neurons, as in spinal cord injury (SCI), may allow the muscle spindle to function without being triggered by the central nervous system, and this can result in spasticity – an exaggerated contraction response to stretch. Hypertonicity can cause contractures, which in turn may cause shortened muscles on one side of the joint and overstretching of the opposing muscle group. To restore balance, stretching exercises for the shortened muscles and strengthening exercises for the opposing muscles should be performed. An assessment will identify tight muscle groups and joints with an imbalance between agonist and antagonist muscles.

Spasms, or involuntary muscle contractions, are common in persons with neurological impairment (*e.g.,* SCI, CP, MS). While flexibility is vital to maintaining muscle length, stretching may induce a spasm; be careful not to force a stretch during a muscle spasm. Flexibility exercises should always be performed within the joint's capacity and may require assistance to achieve the desired ROM. Gradual improvments in flexibility can be achieved over time. Stretch spastic muscle groups, but don't overstretch.

Stretching can be achieved using several methods:

Figure 13.1

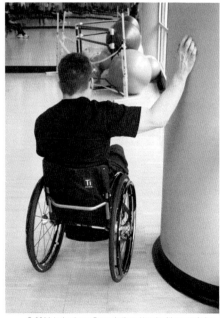

- Passive ROM (PROM) requires full assistance to move the joint through the full desired and functional ROM. Assistance can be provided either manually, by the CIFT, or an assistive device. A band or towel can assist in passive stretching, as can leaning against a wall (see Figure 13.1). The key determinant of passive stretching is that a force other than the muscle itself accomplishes the stretch. A trainer providing passive stretching to a client should be highly trained in safe delivery, as a person with diminished sensation may not be able to provide feedback on limits. Unsafe limits can cause injury to the muscle, tendon, and joint. Communication is essential between trainer and client.
- Active assisted ROM (AAROM) requires a partner to assist in achieving the desired ROM, but also relies on

the muscles ability to produce a portion of the stretch. Training and communication are still essential for safe Active Assisted ROM.

- Active ROM (AROM) requires no assistance but does necessitate active contraction of the opposing muscle being stretched.
- Static stretching, held for 20-30 seconds and in a slow, controlled manner, is most appropriate for flexibility gains, unless specific sport skills are a goal and the client is capable of quicker, more dynamic stretching.

Balance

Adequate balance and balance self-efficacy allows for safe ambulation and movement for daily activities. Reduction in balance poses increased challenges in movement which increases the risk of falling and injury. Loss of the ability to balance can occur suddenly, as in traumatic injury, as the result of progressive conditions, and sometimes due to a lack of attention to balance training.

Impairments resulting from disease or injury (*e.g.,* CP, TBI, MS) or those causing structural changes in the body, as in amputation may affect balance, as will asymmetrical function in limbs and muscles, such as hemiplegia. Wheelchair users may experience balance challenges when transferring or performing ADLs so seated balance exercises can be performed to decrease the risk of injury.

The ability to balance is controlled by three systems of the body:

(1) The somatosensory system is located in receptors in the skin, and provides a sense or feeling of activity and a kinesthetic awareness of body position and movement. When surfaces are stable and smooth, this system is called on primarily to make any necessary adjustments in muscle recruitment. Individuals with decreased sensation or loss of muscle function will have difficulty in utilizing this system for balance.

Figure 13.2. Person with cerebral palsy doing seated balance exercise.

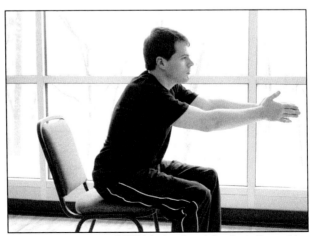

(2) The visual system calls upon the relationship of the head and eyes to surrounding objects and is the primary system used when surfaces become unstable. It becomes faulty in the dark or with advancing age, and is challenged in persons with disabilities or impairments that affect vision.

(3) The vestibular system is activated with head position changes and is located in the inner ear. Many medications and numerous vestibular diseases affect it.

A comprehensive training program will challenge all three systems and should be an integral component of the overall exercise program. Functional assessment of balance will identify the client's comfort and ability to perform seated or standing balance exercises (see Figures 13.2, and 13.3) and is best combined with an educational, problem-solving approach to balance and coordination challenges. Improved balance may also aid in the progression of resistance and cardiovascular exercises, as the client can maintain better control and stability.

Balance exercises can be performed in a standing or seated position. The seated position may be used initially for a client with poor balance and progress to exercises in the standing position. The ultimate goal of balance training is to make movement more functional and decrease the client's risk of falling. This can be achieved by teaching the client to identify the most stable position, to sense imbalance, and by teaching to react and recover from imbalance and recover from a fall.

Figure 13.3

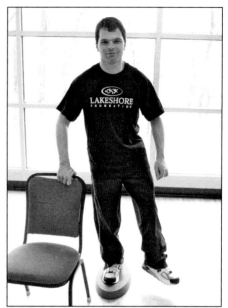

© 2011 Lakeshore Foundation. Used with permission.

Person with cerebral palsy doing standing balance exercise.

References

1. Bryant, Cedric X., & Green, Daniel J. (Eds.). (2003). ACE Personal Trainer Manual: The ultimate Resource for Fitness Professionals (3rd ed.). San Diego, CA: American Council on Exercise.

2. Chen EW, Fu AS, Chan KM, Tsang WW. The effects of Tai Chi on the balance control of elderly persons with visual impairment: a randomised clinical trial. Age Ageing. 2012 Mar;41(2):254-9. Epub 2011 Dec 16.

3. Jankowicz-Szymanska A, Mikolajczyk E, Wojtanowski W. The effect of physical training on static balance in young people with intellectual disability. Res Dev Disabil. 2012 Mar-Apr;33(2):675-81. Epub 2011 Dec 18.

4. National Center on Health, Physical Activity and Disability. (n.d.). Use of the International Classification of Functioning, Disability and Health (ICF) to Prepare Individualized Exercise Prescriptions for People with Disabilities. Retrieved January 06, 2012, from http://www.ncpad.org/fitt/fact_sheet.php?sheet=459

5. Reuter I, Mehnert S, Leone P, Kaps M, Oechsner M, Engelhardt M. Effects of a flexibility and relaxation programme, walking, and nordic walking on Parkinson's disease. J Aging Res. 2011;2011:232473. Epub 2011 Mar 30.

6. Schmid AA, Van Puymbroeck M, Altenburger PA, Dierks TA, Miller KK, Damush TM, Williams LS. Balance and balance self-efficacy are associated with activity and participation after stroke: a cross-sectional study in people with chronic stroke. Arch Phys Med Rehabil. 2012 Jun;93(6):1101-7. Epub 2012 Apr 11.

7. Thompson, Walter R., Bushman, Barbara A., Desch, Julie, & Kravitz, Len. (Eds.). (2010). ACSM's Resources for the Personal Trainer (3rd ed.). Philadelphia, PA: Lippincott Williams & Wilkins.

8. Winnick, Joseph P. (Ed.). (2000). Adapted Physical Education and Sport (3rd ed.). Champaign, IL: Human Kinetics.

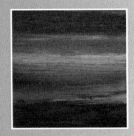

CHAPTER 14

Resistance
Training Programs

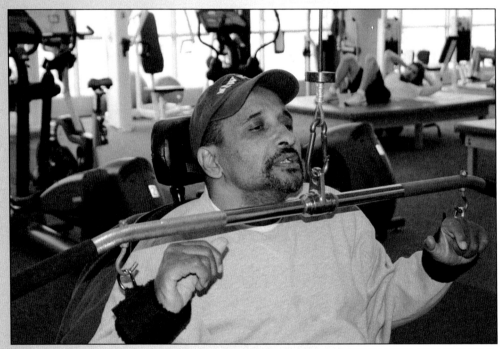

© 2011 Lakeshore Foundation. Used with permission.

The 2008 *Physical Activity Guidelines for Individuals with Disabilities* specify the need for muscle-strengthening activities of moderate or high intensity that involve all major muscle groups on at least two days/week. This is a minimum guideline, required in order for the client to experience muscular strength and endurance gains. Program design should follow the basic principles of overload, progression and mode appropriate for the individual, and is ultimately dependent on the amount of functional muscle mass of the client, availability of accessible equipment, and the creative use of existing equipment. Once a functional assessment has been completed, and S.M.A.R.T. goals have been developed, program design by the CIFT and the client should address exercise choices that focus on reaching goals.

Muscle function can be classified as completely functional, partially functional (paresis) and non-functional (paralysis). All active muscle groups should be trained for each of the groups' potential, and most importantly, within its current ability. With regard for realistic goals and safety, the CIFT should implement "whatever works" for the client. Consistent monitoring of health status, disease status, participant feedback, and short term goal attainment will enhance the credibility of the CIFT and promote the client's independence and feeling of success. Some clients may experience tremendous gains, while some with progressive and remitting conditions may experience less pronounced gains or periodic declines. A special relationship based on professionalism, trust, and openness is important to the success of the client's program.

Increases in strength are achieved with intensities of 80% to 90% 1RM with multiple sets of no more than five to seven repetitions. Training at heavy loads is most safely performed with a partner or assistant, and is appropriate for some individuals with disability that have progressed to an appropriate level and do not have medical contraindications (*e.g.,* high BP, fatigue). Strength routines are especially important for wheelchair users that must regularly transfer their own body weight. Muscular endurance training program design includes intensities of 65% or less 1RM with multiple sets of 8 to 20 repetitions. Muscular endurance routines are appropriate for most beginners and any individuals with contraindications to heavy loads. An intensity near 75% 1RM will provide for strength and endurance increases and is appropriate for many with careful progression. Rest duration between exercises and sets is another variable that can be manipulated to achieve overload and progression. Heavy loads require longer rest between sets while lighter loads require less rest. A decrease in rest duration may be appropriate as strength and endurance gains increase.

When training intensity has been established, exercise selection becomes the key choice in addressing client needs, goals, and movement capabilities. Balanced strength of agonist and antagonist muscle groups is essential for preventing injury, overuse, and for maintaining optimal range of movement and good body alignment. Many wheelchair users overdevelop anterior or pushing muscles (*e.g.,* pec major, anterior deltoids, pec minor) with accompanying weakness in posterior or pulling muscles. Spasticity can provoke muscle imbalance as it habitually places the limb in a position that shortens the muscle on one side of the joint while lengthening the opposing muscle. Over time, the imbalance can cause or exacerbate contractures. Reciprocal inhibition allows for coordinated movement by relaxation of muscles on one side of a joint to accommodate contraction on the other. Approach resistance training of spastic muscles carefully and focus more on opposing muscles.

Single joint exercises isolate a particular muscle or group by requiring movement from only one joint, and while they can strengthen specific muscles, they are not particularly functional. They are, however, appropriate for individuals that may find success with more simple movement and allow for maintaining balance and proper technique. Multi-joint exercises require movement at two or more joints and can mimic activities of daily living, sports skills, and increase function. When incorporating single and multi-joint exercises in a training session, it is recommended to begin with multi-joint activities that utilize several muscle groups simultaneously. Performing single joint movements first can fatigue those muscles needed for later multi-joint movements.

Unilateral exercise, performed by one side, can be useful when motor control is unequal (*e.g.*, hemiplegia, hemiparesis) or when balance impairment makes unilateral exercise more appropriate. Bilateral exercise, utilizing both sides of the body to perform an exercise incorporates more core or torso strength than unilateral exercise. The functional mass of the client will dictate which regimen is more appropriate for goal attainment.

Core strengthening should be included in all exercise programs. Weakness in the core muscles from the neck to the hips can jeopardize the safety and effectiveness of the overall exercise program. Examples of seated core exercises include recline curl, seated waist twist, and knee lifts with crunch.

Strength training equipment can be classified into three general categories (see figures 14.1-3): (1) machines, (2) free weights, and (3) bands, tubing, and manual resistance. Machines provide the greatest stabilization and postural support, but require less recruitment of stabilizing and assister muscles. The accessibility of some machines is limited for persons that cannot transfer. However, several equipment manufacturers have designed machines with roll away seats, making them accessible for a person in a wheelchair to pull directly up to the machine.

Machines do not offer a high degree of functional training and may require bilateral movement, which may not be appropriate for individuals with hemiplegic or hemiparetic conditions. However, machines do offer a higher degree of safety, are easier to use and provide stability for individuals with impaired motor control and balance.

Figure 14.1. Person with quadriplegia doing chest press on Upper Tone machine equipped with specialized wrist support.

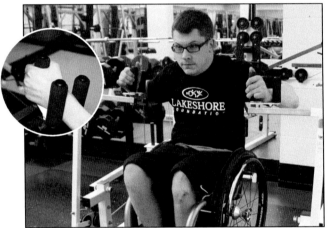

Figure 14.2. Person with quadriplegia exercising with kettlebell.

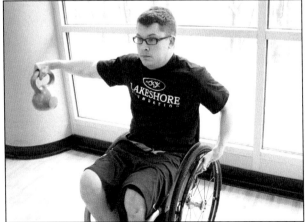

Free weight exercises can be designed to mimic daily functional activities and sport movements, and require multijoint involvement. Free weight exercises are preferred for increased function, but require coordination, skill and balance. Use of free weights may be a progression from machines, and should be encouraged and performed when possible.

Other tools for resistance training such as tubing, stretch bands, and medicine balls, allow for more functional movements than machines. However, they require more skill and an understanding of proper attachment points and orientation of the exercising limb(s) to the attachment. For clients with reduced hand function a number of options are available, such as medicine balls with handles and tubing with ankle and/or wrist Velcro® cuffs. These allow for a variety of activity options. The CIFT should be skilled in using these versatile tools as they can be used limitlessly to add and adapt to resistance-training programs. It is also essential to have items such as gloves, grips, handles, and ACE® bandages available to assist with adaptation of exercises.

Figure 14.3

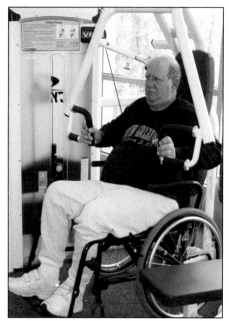

© 2011 Lakeshore Foundation. Used with permission.

Selectorized equipment with removable seat for wheelchair user.

References

1. Bryant, Cedric X., & Green, Daniel J. (Eds.). (2003). ACE Personal Trainer Manual: The Ultimate Resource for Fitness Professionals (3rd ed.). San Diego, CA: American Council on Exercise.

2. Durstine, J. Larry, Moore, Geoffery E., Painter, Patricia, L., & Roberts, Scott O. (Eds.). (2009). ACSM's Exercise Management for Persons with Chronic Diseases and Disabilities (3rd ed.). Champaign, IL: Human Kinetics.

3. Hicks AL, Martin Ginis KA, Pelletier CA, Ditor DS, Foulon B, Wolfe DL. The effects of exercise training on physical capacity, strength, body composition and functional performance among adults with spinal cord injury: a systematic review. Spinal Cord. 2011 Nov;49(11):1103-27. doi: 10.1038/sc.2011.62. Epub 2011 Jun 7.

4. Hill TR, Gjellesvik TI, Moen PM, Tørhaug T, Fimland MS, Helgerud J, Hoff J. Maximal strength training enhances strength and functional performance in chronic stroke survivors. Am J Phys Med Rehabil. 2012 May;91(5):393-400.

5. Jacobs PL. Effects of resistance and endurance training in persons with paraplegia. Med Sci Sports Exerc. 2009 May;41(5):992-7.

6. Lee MJ, Kilbreath SL, Singh MF, Zeman B, Davis GM. Effect of progressive resistance training on muscle performance after chronic stroke. Med Sci Sports Exerc. 2010 Jan;42(1):23-34.

7. Miller, Patricia D., (Ed.). (1995). Fitness Programming and Physical Disability. Champaign, IL: Human Kinetics.

8. National Center on Health, Physical Activity and Disability (n.d.). Resistance Training for Persons with Physical Disabilities. Retrieved January 06, 2012, from http://www.ncpad.org/exercise/fact_sheet.php?sheet=107

9. Sherrill, Claudine., (Ed.). (1998). Adapted Physical Activity, Recreation, and Sport: Crossdisciplinary and Lifespan. (5th ed.). Boston, MA: McGraw-Hill.

10. Thorpe D. The role of fitness in health and disease: status of adults with cerebral palsy. Dev Med Child Neurol. 2009 Oct;51 Suppl 4:52-8.

11. Valent L, Dallmeijer A, Houdijk H, Talsma E, van der Woude L. The effects of upper body exercise on the physical capacity of people with a spinal cord injury: a systematic review. Clin Rehabil. 2007 Apr;21(4):315-30.

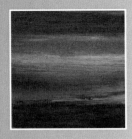

CHAPTER 15

Cardiopulmonary Training Programs

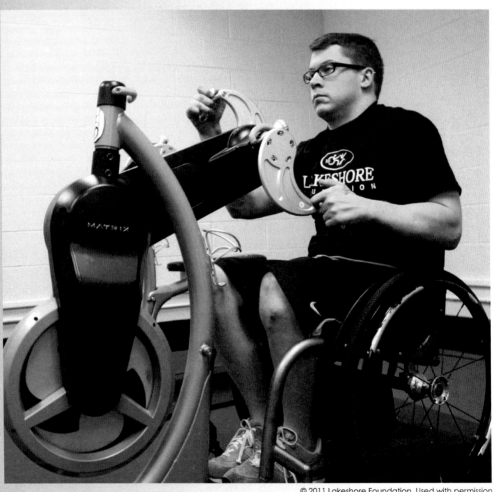

The 2008 *Physical Activity Guidelines for Individuals with Physical Disabilities*, released by the U.S. Department of Health and Human Services, includes a strong statement regarding the importance of regular cardiovascular conditioning for all Americans, including those with physical disabilities. This is the first emphasis of its kind, and clearly outlines recommendations for the intensity and duration of cardiovascular training. Guidelines include aerobic activity for ≥150 minutes/week (moderate intensity) or 75 minutes (vigorous intensity) or equivalent combination. This activity can be performed in episodes of ≥10 minutes and spread throughout the week. Improvements in aerobic capacity will be achieved with these levels of training and are essential for increased heart and lung function. Lowered blood pressure and cholesterol levels may also be a direct result of cardiovascular conditioning.

Improved aerobic capacity will help to control weight, as obesity is of major concern for persons with disabilities due to an increase in sedentary.[9] An analysis of data from the 2001 and 2003 *Behavioral Risk Factor Surveillance Surveys*[8] found that people with disabilities reported a 59% higher rate of obesity (BMI >30) compared to people without disabilities.[4] Data from the *National Health Interview Survey* showed that the prevalence of obesity and morbid obesity (BMI >40) is significantly higher among Caucasians and African Americans with disabilities than those without disabilities, with the morbid obesity rate approximately four times higher.[4] Furthermore, lower rates of physical activity in persons with disabilities aligned with the higher rates of obesity in both racial groups.[4] Other benefits of training are increases in the ability to perform ADL, decreases in depression and anxiety, and an enhancement in the feeling of well-being.

The role of the CIFT is to identify appropriate intensity levels for an initial exercise program and ensure progression that is individualized to the client with a disability. The principles of overload, progression, specificity, and goal setting are essential in safe and effective exercise programming. The CIFT should monitor the client's response to exercise using one of several methods: heart rate, rating of perceived exertion, or the talk test.

Heart rate (HR) training utilizes estimations of maximal heart rate, and training heart rate zones are based on age. Heart rate is widely used in determining training intensity and may be appropriate for many individuals with a disability; however, certain conditions and medications can compromise accuracy. Heart rate response may be altered due to an impairment of the autonomic nervous system (ANS), such as a high level spinal cord injury or multiple sclerosis. Beta blockers (a type of pharmaceutical commonly prescribed for hypertension) will alter the maximum, exercise, and resting heart rate. A person with impaired coordination may have difficulty taking a pulse during exercise, making this method frustrating.

The "talk test" is the simplest method to use for those without speech impairment, as it refers to the client's ability to verbally respond to someone during training. Speech that is uncomfortable (gasping for breath) is an indication the exercise is too challenging and should be decreased. Someone who is too chatty may need to increase the intensity since the goal is to exercise close to the point at which speech becomes difficult.

The rating of perceived exertion (RPE) scale is a subjective measure of the client's overall feeling of exertion and is an optional measure of intensity for those whom HR training is ineffective. Various numeric charts are available, and the client can be asked to respond verbally, with a point of the finger, nod of the head, or blink of the eyes as to which 'intensity' level they are currently exercising at.

Exercise duration should progress toward the recommended level of aerobic activity; ≥150 minutes/week (moderate intensity) or 75 minutes (vigorous intensity) or equivalent combination, performed in episodes of ≥10 minutes and spread throughout the week. It is important, however, to work slowly toward these guidelines. Exercise sessions can begin with short bouts of 10 minutes and can be divided into several sessions until the client can achieve the recommended level. Close monitoring and reference to short and long term goals will add to the client's feeling of success and achievement, thereby increasing adherence.

Modes of Cardiovascular Training

Figure 15.1

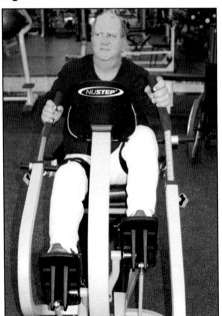

Person with paraplegia using NuStep with leg stabilizers.

Chosen modes of cardiovascular activity will be dictated by the functional ability of the client. A treadmill may not be a safe choice for a client with balance issues, whereas other cardiovascular exercise choices offer a safe and effective mode of training. If a treadmill is appropriate, choose one that offers a slow starting speed (fractions of 1 mph) and always attach the safety strap. A recumbent bicycle provides more stability than an upright bicycle ergometer. Select equipment for both upper and lower body exercise such as a NuStep® Recumbent Cross Trainer (Figure 15.1) or a SciFit® Total Body Elliptical. For the NuStep® trainer, leg stabilizers provide support that keep the user's legs in neutral alignment and WellGrip® handgrips help users with hand and wrist limitations gain the benefits of available upper body exercise. Krankcycle® (Figure 15.2) is a new upper body "spin type" exercise offering an inclusive class setting that satisfies the training needs of participants of all fitness levels and abilities. Exercises on the Krankcycle® can be performed while seated or standing. A removable seat allows wheelchair access. Independent crank arms provide greater variety of movement, and individual control of speed and resistance allows each participant to exercise at their chosen intensity. The adjustable arm crank height and asynchronous design of the Krankcycle® encourages greater range of muscle activation and neuromuscular adaptation.

Utilizing different types of circuit, interval and cross training can increase adherence and motivation by offering choices and options for progression. It is important for an exerciser with a disability, as is true for any regular exerciser, to experience various modes of exercise to diminish monotony and boredom, as well as to prevent overuse injuries. Interval training, using various intensities of work/rest can be achieved with any of the aforementioned equipment choices, and by programming circuit training, alternating between strength and cardio stations, aerobic intensity can be sustained throughout the workout.

Figure 15.2

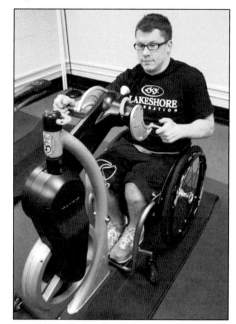

© 2011 Lakeshore Foundation. Used with permission.

Krankcycle with seat removed for wheelchair user.

References

1. Brurok B, Helgerud J, Karlsen T, Leivseth G, Hoff J.Effect of aerobic high-intensity hybrid training on stroke volume and peak oxygen consumption in men with spinal cord injury.Am J Phys Med Rehabil. 2011 May;90(5):407-14.

2. National Center on Health, Physical Activity and Disability. (n.d.). Before & After Fitness Center Makeover. Retrieved January 6, 2012, from http://www.ncpad.org/get/fitnessCenter/index.html

3. National Center on Health, Physical Activity and Disability. (n.d.). Ergometers and Exercise Cycles. Retrieved January 06, 2012, from http://www.ncpad.org/exercise/fact_sheet.php?sheet=5

4. Rimmer, J. A., Wang, E., Yamaki, K., & Davis, B. (2009). Documenting disparities in obesity and disability. FOCUS Technical Brief (24). Austin, TX: SEDL.

5. Semanik PA, Chang RW, Dunlop DD.Aerobic activity in prevention and symptom control of osteoarthritis. PM R. 2012 May;4(5 Suppl):S37-44.

6. Stoller O, de Bruin ED, Knols RH, Hunt KJ. Effects of cardiovascular exercise early after stroke: systematic review and meta-analysis. BMC Neurol. 2012 Jun 22;12(1):45. [Epub ahead of print]

7. Thorpe D. The role of fitness in health and disease: status of adults with cerebral palsy. Dev Med Child Neurol. 2009 Oct;51 Suppl 4:52-8.

8. U.S. Centers for Disease Control and Prevention (2006). 2006 Disability and Health State Chartbook: Profiles of Health for Adults with Disabilities. Atlanta, GA: U.S. Department of Health and Human Services, Author.

9. U.S. Department of Health and Human Services. Office of Disease Prevention and Health Promotion. Healthy People 2020. Washington, DC. Retrieved January 10, 2012, from http://www.healthypeople.gov/2020/topicsobjectives2020/overview.aspx?topicid=9

10. Walter R., Bushman, Barbara A., Desch, Julie, & Kravitz, Len. (Eds.). (2010). ACSM's Resources for the Personal Trainer (3rd ed.). Philadelphia, PA: Lippincott Williams & Wilkins.

Section V

Disability
Awareness

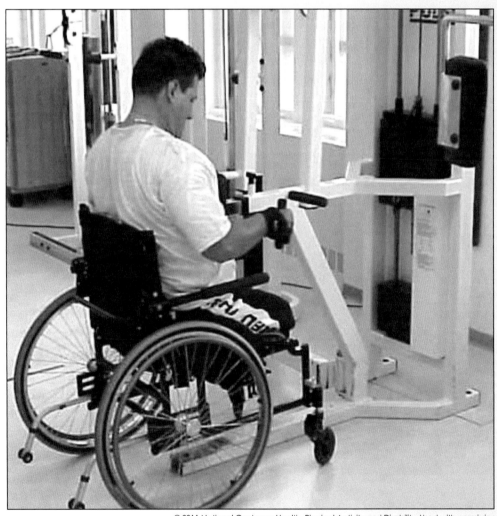

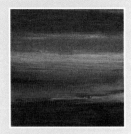

CHAPTER 16

Barriers to
Participation

By Meg Ann Traci, Ph.D.,

Meg Ann Traci is a Research Associate Professor at The University of Montana Rural Institute: Center for Excellence in Disabilities Education, Research, and Services.

Healthy People 2020's (HP2020) Topic Area on *Disability and Health* focuses on the significantly lower rates of participation in everyday life activities among persons with disabilities. Its objectives direct public health agencies to address environmental barriers, including architectural barriers, organizational policies and practices, discrimination, and social attitudes.[15] HP2020's Disability and Health framework and objectives build on the U.S. Surgeon General's "Improving the Health and Wellness of Persons with Disabilities: A Call to Action," which was released in July of 2005 and encouraged:

- Health care providers to see and treat the whole person, not just the disability;
- Educators to teach about disability;
- A public to see an individual's abilities, not just his or her disability; and
- A community to ensure accessible health care and wellness services for persons with disabilities.[16]

The United Nations' Convention on the Rights of Persons with Disabilities,[14] signed by the United States on July 30, 2009 (U.S. ratification still pending), outlines international actions to remove barriers experienced by the 650 million people living with disabilities worldwide. The Convention is framed within a social-ecological model of disability that focuses intervention efforts on societal barriers and prejudices to reduce the experience of disability and limitation.

Most recently, the U.S. Department of Health and Human Services' Office on Minority Health[19] published its "Action Plan to Reduce Racial and Ethnic Health Disparities" and a companion document, the "National Stakeholder Strategy for Achieving Health Equity."[20] Both reports direct coordinated partnership efforts to address health disparities and achieve health equity, some of which include actions and strategies to remove environmental barriers. The National Partnership for Action to End Health Disparities' Federal Interagency Health Equity Team (FIHET) and HP2020 defined health disparity and health equity as follows:

> Health disparity is a particular type of health difference that is closely linked with social, economic, and/or environmental disadvantage. Health disparities adversely affect groups of people who have systematically experienced greater obstacles to health based on their racial and/or ethnic group; religion; socioeconomic status; gender; age; mental health; cognitive, sensory, or physical disability; sexual orientation or gender identity; geographic location; or other characteristics historically linked to discrimination or exclusion.[19, 20]

Health equity is attainment of the highest level of health for all people. Achieving health equity requires valuing everyone equally with focused and ongoing societal efforts to address avoidable inequalities, historical and contemporary injustices, and the elimination of health and healthcare disparities.[19, 20]

Disparities Suggest Barriers

For persons with disabilities, regular physical activity is essential to maintain good health and prevent secondary health conditions associated with sedentary lifestyles. Yet major environmental barriers prevent persons with disabilities from fully participating in physical activity. According to HP2020's Topic Area on *Physical Activity*, in 2008, only 11% of adults with disabilities met the HP2020 physical activity objectives for aerobic physical activity and for muscle-strengthening activity compared to 20% of adults without disabilities (HP2020 Physical Activity Objective 2.4). The percentage of adults with disabilities who engaged in aerobic physical activity was approximately 75% lower compared to the percentage of adults without disabilities, regardless of the level of activity. In other words, about a quarter of adults with disabilities (27%) engaged in moderate aerobic physical activity (HP 2020 Physical Activity Objective 2.1)* compared to about a half of adults without disabilities (47%); and nearly a fifth of adults with disabilities (17%) engaged in intense physical activity (HP2020 Physical Activity Objective 2.2)†

---

* More than 150 min per week of moderate aerobic physical activity or more than 75 min per week of vigorous aerobic physical activity, or an equivalent combination.

† More than 300 min per week of moderate aerobic physical activity or more than 150 min per week of vigorous aerobic physical activity, or an equivalent combination.

Figure 1. Percentages of adult Americans with and without disabilities meeting HP2020 Physical Activity Objectives

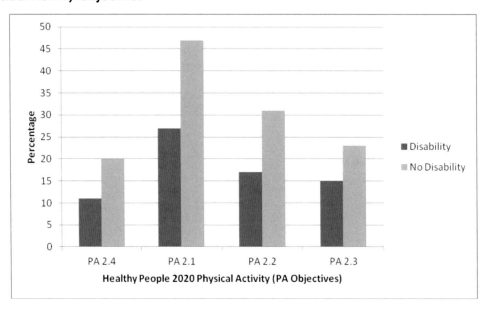

**Figure 2. Rationale for the design
          of a universal instrument that meets
          the needs of all populations**

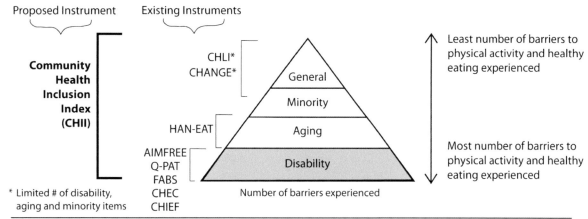

Existing Instruments: *CHLI*-Community Healthy Living Index, *CHANGE*-Community Health aNd Group Evaluation, *HAN-EAT*-Healthy Aging Network Environmental Audit Tool, *AIMFREE*-Accessibility Instruments Measuring Fitness and Recreation Environments, *Q-PAT*- Quick Pathways Accessibility Tool, *FABS*-Facilitators and Barriers Survey, *CHEC*- The Community Health Environment Checklist, *CHIEF*- Craig Hospital Inventory of Environmental Factors.

compared to nearly a third of adults without disabilities (31%). Muscle strengthening activities were performed by nearly a sixth of adults with disabilities (15%) on two or more days of the week (HP2020 Physical Activity Objective 2.3) in 2008 compared to nearly a fourth of adults without disabilities (23%).[15] See *Figure 1* for health disparities that may indicate the more frequent experience of barriers among adults with disabilities compared to adults without disabilities.[9]

Understanding Barriers Experienced by Persons with Disabilities

Persons with disabilities may experience the same barriers that confront most Americans, while also experiencing barriers uniquely contributing to their disability experience, as shown in *Figure 2*.[2] *Figure 2* includes a pyramid with four tiers, each depicting relative numbers of barriers measured by four types of community assessment tools designed to evaluate environments for physical activity and/or healthy eating resources. Generic community assessment tools (*e.g.*, the Community Healthy Living Index) are shown at the top of the pyramid and include relatively few items on barriers to community resources for physical activity and healthy eating as compared to the number of items in tools designed to identify environmental barriers confronting persons with disabilities (*e.g.*, the AIMFREE), which are shown at the bottom of the pyramid.

The pyramid in *Figure 2* conveys how barriers can accumulate for individuals belonging to one or more groups. Individuals may be from communities with relatively few physical activity and healthy eating resources (*e.g.*, rural communities with limited options), may belong to minority and aging groups without access to cultural- or age-appropriate resources, and/or may experience disability without access to inclusionary resources (*e.g.*, a lack of policies promoting staff disability awareness and sensitivity) or accessible options (*e.g.*, see Chapter 4 on the Americans with Disabilities Act (ADA) and Title III, which ensures that both publicly and privately owned fitness and recreation facilities are required to be architecturally accessible to persons with disabilities in areas such as parking, access routes, and restrooms). Finally, the rationale illustrated in *Figure 2* for comprehensive or universal environmental assessments is worth noting. As a part of system improvements, fitness professionals can help identify opportunities to remove barriers confronting persons with disabilities (*e.g.*, a lack of accessible fitness equipment or equipment with universal design features) and to improve the accessibility and inclusionary aspects of fitness centers and recreational facilities.

Adhering to the Physical Activity Guidelines

The "2008 Physical Activity Guidelines for Americans" are for all Americans. The Guidelines provide two additional recommendations to improve accessibility and inclusion: (1) consult a health care provider about the Guidelines and how disabilities can affect physical activity options; and (2) seek advice from professionals with knowledge about physical activity and disability who can help develop a physical activity routine (*e.g.*, fitness professionals) (see Chapter 7: Additional Considerations for Some Adults http://www.health.gov/PAGuidelines/ guidelines/chapter7.aspx). While these recommendations are helpful, persons with disabilities may experience barriers when following either recommendation. The first recommendation suggests a consultation between an individual and a health care provider who is knowledgeable on disability, the Guidelines, and on possible adaptations that will yield health promoting benefits for persons with disabilities. This knowledge also involves an understanding of the rights of persons with disabilities as well as a respect for varying cultures, lifestyles, values, and age groups.[4, 6] Staff at local rehabilitation hospitals, service agencies, or at centers for independent living can assist individuals to find qualified health care professionals who can help them understand the Guidelines. Resources are available that support persons with disabilities to advocate effectively for quality care with their health care professional(s) such as, "You and Your Doctor: A Short Guide To Your Rights And Responsibilities."[12] The Guideline's second recommendation encourages persons with disabilities to seek professionals who can help them modify specific fitness and physical activities to match abilities and interests, and who can support them in their physical activity routines as needed (*e.g.*, weight lifting). Only a limited number of qualified fitness professionals are available to persons with disabilities who are attempting to follow this recommendation; however, the number is growing. The expertise of these professionals may need to be promoted for broader access within communities. Also, there are payment and reimbursement models that address cost barriers associated with a fitness professional that need to be explored and promoted further by persons with disabilities and disability service organizations.

Overcoming Barriers to Physical Activity

The U.S. Centers for Disease Control and Prevention's (CDC) guidance, "Overcoming Barriers to Physical Activity,"[17] reviews common barriers to physical activity and suggests strategies for addressing them. In general, the CDC's guidance provides a good starting point, but a greater understanding of how barriers are experienced by persons with disabilities is needed to support effective action steps for fitness clients with disabilities. For example, the CDC guidance provides the following suggestions for addressing the 'lack of time' barrier to physical activity:

- Identify available time slots.
- Monitor your daily activities for one week.
- Identify at least three 30 minute time slots you could use for physical activity.
- Add physical activity to your daily routine. For example, walk or ride your bike to work or shopping, organize school activities around physical activity, walk the dog, exercise while you watch TV, park farther away from your destination, etc. Select activities requiring minimal time, such as walking, jogging, or stair climbing.[17]

Implementing these strategies may require considerations and efforts for a person with a disability that are beyond what might be required for someone without a disability. In an early study, researchers[5,7] found 6 of 27 barriers experienced by persons with physical disability accessing a health promotion program at centers for independent living (facilities that are physically accessible) to be most problematic: (1) Fatigue ("I tire easily"); (2) Pain ("I have pain when I do too much"); (3) Disability ("My disability limits me too much these days"); (4) Need for assistance ("I will need someone to help me"); (5) Control of body functions ("I could lose control over my bowel/bladder"); and (6) Transportation ("I don't have accessible transportation"). Their findings inform possible modifications to the CDC's above suggestions. For example, persons with disabilities may have fewer available time slots for physical activity within a complex schedule of other health maintenance behaviors, including behaviors for preventing secondary health conditions and activities of daily living. The physical activity may be less efficiently performed because of a lack of adequate assistive technology or personal assistance supports (*e.g.*, sleeping, personal hygiene, dressing, eating, pain management, bowel/bladder routines). With fewer options available, identifying a time slot for physical activity may mean forgoing some other meaningful life activity. In addition, schedule change(s) may require persons with disabilities to coordinate or rearrange transportation and supports. To set a schedule, persons with disabilities may also need to consult a health care provider about the appropriate dose and schedule of physical activity suited to their conditions and abilities.

Similarly, persons with disabilities may need to consult a fitness professional to individualize physical activities that are not mobility-dependent and that can be integrated into daily routines (*e.g.,* performing specific daily living tasks at the highest level of independence).

Further Considerations

In a series of national focus groups, Rimmer, Riley, Wang, Rauworth and Jurkowski[11] gathered information on physical activity barriers facing persons with disabilities. Four focus groups were held in 10 cities. Each focus group included either persons with disabilities, architects, fitness/recreation professionals, or city planners and park district managers. All 42 participants with disabilities were limited by a physical condition associated with spinal cord injuries; back problems; and conditions affecting the use of their arms, hands, or legs. The study identified 10 barriers to physical activity: (1) barriers and facilitators related to the built and natural environment; (2) economic issues; (3) emotional and psychological barriers; (4) equipment barriers; (5) barriers related to the use and interpretation of guidelines, codes, regulations, and laws; (6) information related barriers; (7) professional knowledge, education, and training issues; (8) perceptions and attitudes of persons who are not disabled, including professionals; (9) policies and procedures both at the facility and community level; and (10) availability of resources.

Rimmer and his colleagues' work informed the development of the AIMFREE assessment tools,[10] available in both professional and consumer versions. AIMFREE can be used to identify facilitators and barriers at fitness facilities and guide action planning. Fitness professionals can use AIMFREE to acquaint themselves with the range of accessible physical activity options at various fitness and recreational facilities, and to identify options that could be modified for accessibility to a variety of abilities. Fitness professionals can also use AIMFREE to help identify training needs of staff and colleagues; identify areas to improve policies at facilities; and identify environmental changes for which to advocate (See Chapter 6). Fitness professionals might give the AIMFREE consumer version to clients in order to educate them about opportunities and barriers at a facility. Resources and strategies to address other barriers, such as economic, emotional, psychological, and information barriers identified in the study by Rimmer and his colleagues, include peer support and wellness programs, national resources centers, national coalitions (*e.g.,* the Inclusive Fitness Coalition), and local health professionals and community service organizations.

To inform physical activity intervention programs for persons with intellectual disability (ID), Bodde and Seo[1] selected and reviewed seven studies of barriers to physical activity experienced by adults with ID. Many barriers to physical activity that they identified were similar to barriers found in studies of the general population, including financial constraints, lack of support from others, lack of transportation, limited options, limited awareness, and limited access. However, several studies found that unique physical activity barriers also were confronting persons with ID, such as discouragement from physical activity by others for safety reasons; ambiguous policies in home or day program services; and support staff constraints limiting individuals' planning, transportation, and

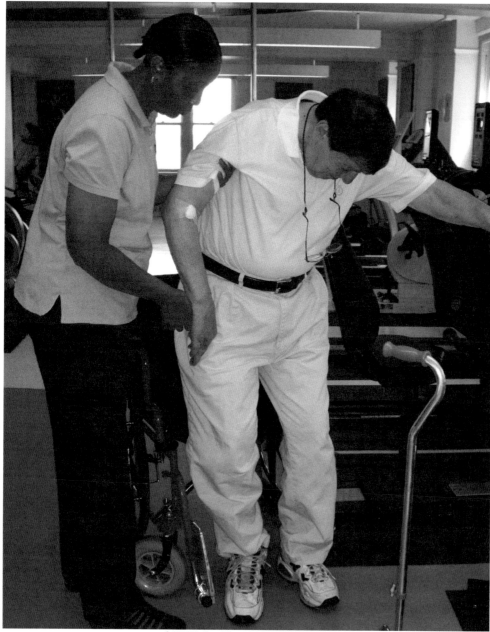

© 2011 National Center on Health, Physical Activity and Disability. Used with permission.

access to written information. Bodde and Seo also indicated that removal of any barrier using service system resources would require sustained advocacy and may take time. For example, inadequate transportation for someone with ID could mean a lack of accessible transportation during needed days and hours, a lack of an individual's knowledge about transportation options and how to use them, and/or a lack of staff support for an individual to access transportation options. Developing physical activity options in the home and integrating walking as alternative transportation into daily routines are seemingly easy solutions for addressing these barriers, but within the context of home and community based service systems, such changes may require hiring new staff, reorganizing others' schedules, and/or changing agency policies. The "2008 Physical Activity Guidelines for Americans" promote (individual level) personal goal setting, which can be a formal process of organizing home and community-based service supports that involves an individual and his or her case manager and personal support team. Providing guidance on appropriate fitness goals and activities to be considered during these types of planning processes may lead to more effective individual supports for persons with disabilities.[13]

Conclusion

Varieties of barriers to physical activity confront individuals with disabilities and contribute systematically to health disparities experienced by populations with disabilities. Some barriers are commonly experienced by many Americans, and some are unique to persons with disabilities. Working with clients with disabilities to address these barriers in their personal lives and in their communities is necessary to support their efforts to be physically active. National initiatives provide frameworks for the fitness industry and its professionals to address environmental barriers and to promote the many benefits of physical activity to persons with disabilities[3] using strategies and tactics that will persuade individuals with disabilities to use their limited resources to become physically active.[8]

Resources
- AIMFREE (Accessibility Instruments Measuring Fitness and Recreation Environments) a multi-dimensional validated instrument that can determine the accessibility of six categories: (1) built environment, (2) equipment, (3) information, (4) policies, (5) swimming pools, and (6) professional behaviors (attitudes and knowledge). Available at www.nchpad.org.
- North Carolina Office on Disability and Health (2001). Removing Barriers to Health Clubs and Fitness Facilities. Chapel Hill, NC: Frank Porter Graham Child Development Center.
- U.S. Access Board, (800) 872-2253 (voice), (800) 993-2822 (TTY), or www.access-board.gov/.
- Active Living by Design. www.activelivingbydesign.org/category/topic/ physical-activity-and-disabilities

References

1. BODDE AE, SEO D. A REVIEW OF SOCIAL AND ENVIRONMENTAL BARRIERS TO PHYSICAL ACTIVITY FOR ADULTS WITH INTELLECTUAL DISABILITIES. DISABILITY AND HEALTH JOURNAL. 2009; 2:57-66.

2. CENTER ON HEALTH PROMOTION RESEARCH FOR PERSONS WITH DISABILITIES. RATIONALE FOR THE DESIGN OF A UNIVERSAL INSTRUMENT THAT MEETS THE NEEDS OF ALL POPULATIONS. UNIVERSITY OF ILLINOIS-CHICAGO, CHICAGO; 2011.

3. COOPER R, QUATRANO L, AXELSON P, HARLAN W, STINEMAN M, FRANKLIN B. RESEARCH ON PHYSICAL ACTIVITY AND HEALTH AMONG PEOPLE WITH DISABILITIES: A CONSENSUS STATEMENT. J REHABIL RES DEV. 1999; 36:142-154.

4. IEZZONI, LI. PUBLIC HEALTH GOALS FOR PERSONS WITH DISABILITIES: LOOKING AHEAD TO 2020. DISABILITY AND HEALTH JOURNAL. 2009; 2:111-115.

5. MURPHY-SOUTWICK C, SEEKINS T. READINESS FOR HEALTH PROMOTION. MISSOULA, MT: RESEARCH AND TRAINING CENTER ON DISABILITY IN RURAL COMMUNITIES, THE UNIVERSITY OF MONTANA; 2000.

6. PETERSON PA, QUARSTEIN VA. DISABILITY AWARENESS TRAINING FOR DISABILITY PROFESSIONALS. DISABIL REHABIL. 2001; 23:43-48.

7. RAVESLOOT, C. RURAL OUTREACH: GETTING THE WORD OUT THAT BRINGS PEOPLE IN. WORKSHOP PRESENTED AT THE ASSOCIATION OF PROGRAMS FOR RURAL INDEPENDENT LIVING ANNUAL CONFERENCE, 2006. SAN ANTONIO, TX.

8. RAVESLOOT C, RUGERIO C, ISPEN C, TRACI MA, RIGLES B, BOEHM T, WARE D, SEEKINS T. HEALTH BEHAVIOR CHANGE IN THE CONTEXT OF THE DISABILITY EXPERIENCE. DISABILITY AND HEALTH JOURNAL. 2011; 4:19-23.

9. RIMMER JH. THE CONSPICUOUS ABSENCE OF PEOPLE WITH DISABILITIES IN PUBLIC FITNESS AND RECREATION FACILITIES: LACK OF INTEREST OR LACK OF ACCESS? AMERICAN JOURNAL OF HEALTH PROMOTION. 2005; 19:327-329, ii.

10. RIMMER JH, RILEY BB, WANG E, RAUWORTH AE. DEVELOPMENT AND VALIDATION OF AIMFREE: ACCESSIBILITY INSTRUMENTS MEASURING FITNESS AND RECREATION ENVIRONMENTS. DISABIL REHABIL. 2004; 26:1087-1095.

11. RIMMER JH, RILEY BB, WANG E, RAUWORTH AE, JURKOWKSI J. PHYSICAL ACTIVITY PARTICIPATION AMONG PERSONS WITH DISABILITIES: BARRIERS AND FACILITATORS. AM J PREV MED. 2004; 26:419-425.

12. REHABILITATION RESEARCH AND TRAINING CENTER ON SPINAL CORD INJURY (2008). YOU AND YOUR DOCTOR: A SHORT GUIDE TO YOUR RIGHTS AND RESPONSIBILITIES. HTTP://WWW.ILRU.ORG/HTML/PUBLICATIONS/SCI/LIBRARY/YOU_AND_YOUR_DOCTOR.PDF . ACCESSED DECEMBER 30, 2011.

13. TRACI MA, SEEKINS T, SZALDA-PETREE AC., RAVESLOOT CH. ASSESSING SECONDARY CONDITIONS AMONG ADULTS WITH DEVELOPMENTAL DISABILITIES: A PRELIMINARY STUDY. MENTAL RETARDATION. 2002; 40: 119-131.

14. UN GENERAL ASSEMBLY, CONVENTION ON THE RIGHTS OF PERSONS WITH DISABILITIES: RESOLUTION / ADOPTED BY THE GENERAL ASSEMBLY, 24 JANUARY 2007, A/RES/61/106. HTTP://WWW.UNHCR.ORG/REFWORLD/DOCID/45F973632.HTML . ACCESSED DECEMBER 31, 2011.

15. U.S. DEPARTMENT OF HEALTH AND HUMAN SERVICES. HEALTHY PEOPLE 2020: IMPROVING THE HEALTH OF AMERICANS. WASHINGTON, DC: USDHHS 2010.

16. U.S. DEPARTMENT OF HEALTH AND HUMAN SERVICES, OFFICE OF THE SURGEON GENERAL. THE 2005 SURGEON GENERAL'S CALL TO ACTION TO IMPROVE THE HEALTH AND WELLNESS OF PERSONS WITH DISABILITIES: CALLING YOU TO ACTION.WASHINGTON, DC: USDHHS; 2005.

17. U.S. DEPARTMENT OF HEALTH AND HUMAN SERVICES, THE CENTERS FOR DISEASE CONTROL AND PREVENTION. OVERCOMING BARRIERS TO PHYSICAL ACTIVITY. WASHINGTON, DC: USDHHS; 2011. HTTP://WWW.CDC.GOV/PHYSICALACTIVITY/EVERYONE/GETACTIVE/BARRIERS.HTML . ACCESSED DECEMBER 31, 2011.

18. U.S. DEPARTMENT OF HEALTH AND HUMAN SERVICES. 2008 PHYSICAL ACTIVITY GUIDELINES FOR AMERICANS. WASHINGTON, DC: USDHHS; 2008. HTTP://WWW.HEALTH.GOV/ PAGUIDELINES/DEFAULT/ASPX . ACCESSED DECEMBER 31, 2011.

19. U.S. DEPARTMENT OF HEALTH AND HUMAN SERVICES. OFFICE ON MINORITY HEALTH. ACTION PLAN TO REDUCE RACIAL AND ETHNIC HEALTH DISPARITIES, WASHINGTON, DC: USDHHS; 2011. HTTP://MINORITYHEALTH.HHS.GOV/NPA/TEMPLATES/CONTENT.ASPX?LVL=1&LVLID=33&ID=285 . ACCESSED DECEMBER 31, 2011.

20. U.S. DEPARTMENT OF HEALTH AND HUMAN SERVICES, OFFICE ON MINORITY HEALTH. NATIONAL STAKEHOLDER STRATEGY FOR ACHIEVING HEALTH EQUITY. WASHINGTON, DC: USDHHS; 2011. HTTP://MINORITYHEALTH.HHS.GOV/NPA/TEMPLATES/CONTENT.ASPX?LVL=1&LVLID=33&ID=286 . ACCESSED DECEMBER 31, 2011.

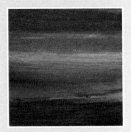

CHAPTER 17

Spinal Cord Lesions

By Susan Ostertag, PT, DPT, NCS; and Molly Blair, CES, CIFT

Susan is an APTA Board Certified Neurological Clinical Specialist and works as a Clinical Assistant Faculty member at the School of Physical Therapy and the University of Montana, where she teaches in the areas of neurological rehabilitation, functional mobility, and interventions. She is the director of the University of Montana Physical Therapy Clinic and the New Directions Wellness Center, which provide physical therapy services and an accessible, assisted fitness center for individuals on campus and from the community. She is also the director of the UM Student Run Clinic, who's mission is to provide wellness services to uninsured patients. Susan has worked as a physical therapist for 19 years and continues to see patients with neurological and other chronic conditions. In addition, Susan participates in a number of community based outreach programs and seminars each year sharing information about neurological rehabilitation, fitness, and the role of physical therapy for chronic disease and disability.

Molly Blair is a Clinical Exercise Specialist, an ACSM/NCHPAD Certified Inclusive Fitness Trainer, as well as the program manager at New Directions. With a Bachelor of Science in Exercise Science from the University of Montana, she has worked with the New Directions Wellness Center for over eight years. She also spent a year working at St. Patrick's Hospital in the Wellness Center as a cardiac rehabilitation aide. Besides her knowledge of how to provide exceptional care for the physically limited, Molly brings the element of charm that keeps clients coming back for more.

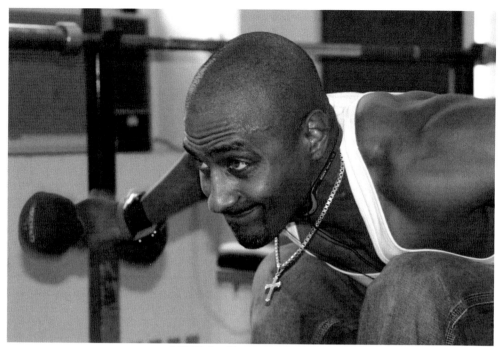

© 2011 National Center on Health, Physical Activity and Disability. Used with permission.

Spinal cord injuries (SCI) acquired due to trauma or illness affects up to 12,000 people per year in the United States.[1] About 80% of the people who sustain SCI are male, and most are between the ages of 16 and 30 years old. These injuries occur primarily as a result of motor vehicles accidents, falls, violence, and sports. Some also occur as a result of illness or surgery.

These injuries have a direct effect on a person's ability to function, as any damage at any point along the spinal cord affects the areas innervated by the descending nerves at or below the level of lesion. The lesion can affect the function of the motor system, sensation, respiratory status, cardiovascular system, gastrointestinal tract, and integumentary system. Injury to the cervical segments (C1-C8) or the highest thoracic segment (T1) causes tetraplegia (or called quadriplegia) with impairment of the arms, trunk, legs, and pelvic organs (bladder, bowels, and sexual organs). Injury to the thoracic segments (T2-T12) causes paraplegia, with impairment to the trunk, legs, pelvic organs, or some combination of these. Injury to the lumbar or sacral segment (L1-L5, S1-S4) results in impairment to the legs or pelvic organs or both. Because of conditions related to body changes, including impaired mobility, dependence on others for functional activities, altered sexual function, and, incontinence of bowel and/or bladder, people with spinal cord injuries may also experience psychosocial difficulties.

The primary injury, or initial SCI, often results in paralysis and a loss of sensation to all or part of the body that is innervated below the level of the lesion. A person with incomplete SCI may have some ability to move or may have some sensation below the level of the injury. A complete SCI will present with both complete sensory and motor loss below the level of lesion. Even though the spinal cord injury is identified by the area where damage occurred, each individual must be assessed to determine the extent of the weakness and loss of sensation.

Individuals that sustain an SCI first undergo spinal shock, which is temporary and occurs after damage to the spinal cord. Upon recovery from the spinal shock, which can last for hours or months, reflex recovery occurs before voluntary movement. Some individuals recover almost to full capacity, and others never regain full function. Neurological return after SCI is dependent upon many factors and refers to regaining the ability to move voluntarily or have a restoration of normal sensation. Return can occur for several years after injury, but is most pronounced in the first three months.

In contrast, abnormal reflexive functioning is not qualified as neurological return. The reflexive recovery eventually becomes spasticity, and is more commonly seen in individuals with incomplete SCI's, as well as cervical and upper thoracic lesions. Spasticity refers to an involuntary increase in muscle tone. It is usually velocity dependent, meaning the faster the motion of the limb the stronger the spasticity. Spasticity can occur in patterns; can vary and depend upon patient and environmental conditions; and may affect function and gait adversely or positively. Spasticity may also increase as a symptom of urinary tract infection, skin breakdown, or when any noxious stimulus is sensed by the body. Benefits of spasticity may include maintaining some level of muscle tone and bone strength and maintaining circulation. Some individuals may use it to assist with functional activities such as standing.

Other systems of the body will require medical consideration. Proper bladder care is needed to prevent urinary tract infections, incontinence, overfilling, and minimize spasticity. The gastrointestinal system may not be functioning, and the patient may require a feeding tube. He or she may also require a scheduled bowel program to avoid incontinence. Skin breakdown is an ever present threat, and must be prevented through proper positioning when seated or lying down with regular pressure reliefs through a change in position every two hours at minimum.

The respiratory and cardiovascular systems are also affected by SCI. The muscles responsible for breathing may not function, and the individual may depend on a respirator for mechanical ventilation, or on use of accessory breathing muscles such as upper trapezius and scalene muscles if the diaphragm, abdominals, and intercostals are not properly functioning.

Cardiovascular considerations are especially noticeable in individuals with SCI lesions above T6. The individuals may experience a drop in heart rate, or a drop in blood pressure called orthostatic hypotension, when attaining an upright position. Orthostatic hypotension is the result of a drop in blood pressure >20 for SBP and >10 for DBP. The individual may be dizzy, nauseated, or light headed and should be repositioned into supine with feet elevated. To help prevent orthostatic hypotension, insure proper hydration and avoid positions that interrupt blood flow.

Autonomic dysreflexia (AD) refers to an abnormal sympathetic response to a noxious stimulus. This can occur very quickly, and can be life threatening. Symptoms of AD include elevated systolic and diastolic blood pressure >20 mmHg than their normal post injury level, headache, slower heart rate than post injury level, profuse sweating, skin flushing, piloerection above level of injury, visual deficits, nasal congestion, anxiety, and cardiac arrhythmias. Immediately place the individual into an upright sitting position to help lower blood pressure, or if already seated remove any potentially noxious stimuli such as full catheter, tight clothing, or other pressure.

Another medical consideration is the risk of developing ectopic bone called heterotrophic ossifications. These can result in limited motion of a joint, severe pain, inflammation, and inability to move a once movable limb. Individuals with SCI are also at risk for development of deep vein thrombosis due to the immobility and lack of muscle contraction following an injury.

Medications commonly prescribed for individuals with SCI lesions include medications to relax or stimulate the bladder muscles, suppositories and laxatives to assist with bowel management, antispasmodic medication to reduce muscle spasms, vasopressors to help maintain blood pressure, antihypertensives to reduce the risk of autonomic dysreflexia symptoms, heparin to reduce the risk of deep vein thrombosis, as well as antidepressives and pain medication. Common side effects of these medications include lethargy, hypotension, nausea, fatigue and even heart palpitations.

Exercise Prescription
For Spinal Cord Injury

The medical issues resulting from damage to the central nervous system, the secondary medical issues, and the medications taken must be considered with any exercise prescription. Close monitoring of blood pressure and heart rate at rest and with activity as well as recovery is indicated. Assess for any signs of autonomic dysreflexia frequently when starting a new activity. Use a Borg Scale to help determine level of exertion, as heart rate levels will not elevate to the preinjury levels with exercise due to nervous system damage and/or medication side effects. For persons with tetraplegia or high-level paraplegia, exercise should take place in a thermoneutral or cool gym with air-conditioning to control temperature.

These individuals are at high risk for injury due to lack of sensation and muscle weakness, and the integumentary system may need to be assessed with any new activity that involves sustained pressure. As the individual may not feel pain, noxious stimulus may present as increased spasticity or with other autonomic dysreflexia type symptoms. Individuals will also be at risk for falling or having balance dysfunction due to the lack of motor control and/or sensation. Trunk straps or other external support should be used when exercising to stabilize the trunk and minimize the risk of falling.

Emphasis should be on strengthening any intact muscles, maintaining and/or gaining muscle length and range of motion, and facilitating recovery of weakened muscles. This includes the abdominals and trunk extensors as well as extremities. To prevent upper extremity overuse syndrome, varying exercise modes, strengthening muscles of the upper back and posterior shoulder, and especially external shoulder rotators are recommended. Stretching muscles is also indicated to reduce spasticity, prevent contractures, and decrease pain. Precautions exist for stretching when the patient requires shorter muscles for functional use, such as the lumbar and trunk extensors for passive trunk stability and the finger and wrist flexors to assist with grasping ("tenodesis"). The American College of Sports Medicine (ACSM) recommends performing 20 to 60 minutes of continuous aerobic exercise or in 10 minutes sessions three to five times per week.

Spina Bifida

According to the Spina Bifida Association, there are an estimated 166,000 people in the United States living with Spina Bifida. Spina Bifida is a neural tube defect that happens when the spinal column doesn't close completely when the fetus is developing. The neurological deficits experienced by the individual will be dependent on the severity of the defect and result in muscle weakness and sensory loss below the level of the defect. The following types of Spina Bifida are identified by the Spina Bifida Association at **http://www.spinabifidaassociation.org/atf/cf**

Occult Spinal Dysraphism (OSD)

The spinal cord may not grow correctly and can cause serious problems as a child grows up. Infants who might have OSD should be followed by a physician.

Spina Bifida Occulta

It is often called "hidden Spina Bifida" because about 15% of healthy people have it and do not know it. Spina Bifida occulta does not cause harm;, has no signs; and, the spinal cord and nerves are fine. People usually learn they have it after having an X-ray of their back.

Meningocele

This condition causes part of the spinal cord to come through the spine, like a sac that is pushed out. Nerve fluid is in the sac, and there is usually no nerve damage. Individuals with this condition may have minor disabilities.

Myelomeningocele (Meningomyelocele)

This is the most severe form of Spina Bifida. It occurs when parts of the spinal cord and nerves come through the open part of the spine. It causes nerve damage and other disabilities. Seventy to ninety percent of children with this condition also have too much fluid on their brains. A shunt may be needed, and these individuals need medical management throughout their lives.

Anyone with a new onset of neurological symptoms should be referred immediately to a physician or emergency room dependent on the severity of the symptoms. Other considerations for individuals with Spina Bifida include the risk of depression, possible learning disabilities, and other developmental disabilities.

About 90% of babies born with Spina Bifida now live to be adults; about 80% have normal intelligence; and, about 75% engage in recreational activities. These individuals are at risk for falls, osteoporosis, and skin breakdown. There is a wide range of weakness and sensation loss that will vary between individuals, so each individual must be assessed prior to exercise instruction. Assessment of spasticity, contractures, balance, cognitive level and safety must also be performed.

Exercise Prescription For Spina Bifida

Individuals with Spina Bifida benefit from exercise for several reasons. A variety of exercise modalities including aerobic, strengthening, and stretching may assist the individual in many ways. The benefits of exercise may include increased independence or safety with functional mobility, improved cardiovascular fitness; and, reduce the risk of developing secondary conditions such as heart disease, osteoporosis, diabetes and obesity.

These individuals may experience a max heart rate that is significantly lower than normal and special considerations should be taken when prescribing an exercise program. Use of RPE, rate of perceived exertion scale, instead of heart rate may be indicated to obtain an accurate assessment of the individual's response to exercise. The ACSM guidelines can be followed to perform 20 to 60 minutes of continuous aerobic exercise or 10 minute bouts three to five times per week. The individuals are at risk for fractures due to the high risk they have for developing osteoporosis during their lifetime. Special consideration must be given to positions and resistance during strength training. Strengthening should be focused on intact muscle groups, 3-5 days/week. Emphasis on upright posture is necessary, and external trunk support or other adaptive straps may be indicated to insure good extremity alignment and safety to prevent injury and falls. Stretching may be indicated as these individuals are at risk for spasticity, contractures, joint pain, joint degeneration due to the muscle weakness and loss of sensation that may result from the Spina Bifida.

Post-Polio Syndrome

According to the National Institute of Neurological Disorders and Stroke, Post-Polio Syndrome (PPS) is a condition that affects polio survivors years after recovery from an initial acute attack of the poliomyelitis virus. PPS is mainly characterized by new weakening in muscles that were previously affected by the polio infection and in muscles that seemingly were unaffected. Symptoms include slowly progressive muscle weakness, unaccustomed fatigue (both generalized and muscular), and, at times, muscle atrophy. Pain from joint degeneration and increasing skeletal deformities such as scoliosis are common. Some patients experience only minor symptoms. While less common, others may develop visible muscle atrophy, or wasting.

According to estimates by the National Center for Health Statistics, more than 440,000 polio survivors in the United States may be at risk for PPS. This condition appears to be related to the degeneration of individual nerve terminals in the motor units that remain after the initial illness. The poliovirus attacks specific neurons in the brainstem and the spinal cord, and may be due to an overuse of the nerve cells that have recovered from the initial polio illness. This syndrome is characterized by a slow, unpredictable course of worsening weakness and decrease in function.

PPS does not have any medications approved for specific treatment of the condition, but these individuals are at risk for development of secondary conditions such as arthritis, heart disease, obesity, diabetes, contractures, and osteoporosis due to decreased strength and mobility. Use of assistive devices may be recommended for improved function, ambulation, completion of activities of daily living, and the prevention of falls. Activities that result in pain or fatigue that lasts more than 10 minutes are not recommended. Education in self pacing of daily activities and exercise is necessary.

Exercise Prescription For Post-Polio Syndrome

According to the National Institute of Health, exercise is safe and effective when carefully implemented. However, persons who have severe atrophic polio and have recent weakness should not exercise. Strength training and aerobic exercise will be most effective in those muscles not affected by the PPS. When starting an exercise program, the individual must work at a low to moderate level of intensity and progress very gradually to prevent joint and tissue damage. Emphasis should be placed on cardiovascular training and endurance exercises. The ACSM guidelines can be followed recommending performing 20 to 60 minutes of continuous aerobic exercise or in 10 minutes sessions three to five times per week. Heavy lifting and strenuous activity should be avoided. An aquatic setting is excellent for individuals with PPS as the water provides a low impact to no impact environment to preserve joint function, and the warmth of the water is beneficial to relaxing muscles and relieving joint pain. Discontinue exercise that results in weakness or prolonged recovery, meaning any fatigue that lasts more than 10 minutes. Stretching exercises may be indicated to help increase range of motion, decrease joint pain, and to decrease the risk of contracture development.

Summary

To help prevent secondary conditions, injury or muscle atrophy while maximizing the individual's functional potential, an individual with traumatic or acquired Spinal Cord Lesions must participate in an exercise program including cardiovascular fitness, strengthening, and flexibility as appropriate for their condition. Each individual should obtain clearance from their primary care provider or any other provider that is treating the neurological condition or injury. The individual should be referred to a professional trainer or health care provider with experience in establishing exercise regimens for individuals with spinal cord conditions and injuries.

Resources

- HTTP://WWW.SPINABIFIDAASSOCIATION.ORG/SITE/C.LIKWL7PLLRF/B.2642297/K.5F7C/ SPINA_BIFIDA_ASSOCIATION.HTM. ACCESSED ON SEPTEMBER 1, 2011.
- HTTP:/WWW.NINDS.NIH.GOV/DISORDERS/POST_POLIO/DETAIL_POST_POLIO.HTM. ACCESSED ON SEPTEMBER 1, 2011.
- HTTP://WWW.NCHPAD.COM/DISABILITY/FACT_SHEET.PHP?SHEET=256 "DISABILITY/CONDITION: SPINA BIFIDA- PHYSICAL ACTIVITY GUIDELINES" ACCESSED ON SEPTEMBER 1, 2011.
- HTTP://WWW.NCHPAD.COM/DISABILITY/FACT_SHEET.PHP?SHEET=130 "DISABILITY/CONDITION: SPINAL CORD INJURY AND EXERCISE" ACCESSED ON SEPTEMBER 1, 2011.
- HTTP://WWW.NCHPAD.COM/DISABILITY/FACT_SHEET.PHP?SHEET=62 "DISABILITY/CONDITION: SPINAL CORD INJURY" ACCESSED ON SEPTEMBER 1, 2011.
- HTTP://WWW.NCHPAD.COM/DISABILITY/FACT_SHEET.PHP?SHEET=63 "DISABILITY/CONDITION: POST POLIOMYELITIS" ACCESSED ON SEPTEMBER 1, 2011.

References

1. SOMERS, M. SPINAL CORD INJURY: FUNCTIONAL REHABILITATION, 3RD ED.. UPPER SADDLE RIVER, NJ: PEARSON EDUCATION, INC, 2010.

2. HTTP://WWW.SPINABIFIDAASSOCIATION.ORG/SITE/C.LIKWL7PLLRF/B.2642297/K.5F7C/SPINA_BIFIDA_ ASSOCIATION.HTM. ACCESSED ON SEPTEMBER 1, 2011.

3. HTTP:/WWW.NINDS.NIH.GOV/DISORDERS/POST_POLIO/DETAIL_POST_POLIO.HTM. ACCESSED ON SEPTEMBER 1, 2011.

4. HTTP://WWW.NCHPAD.COM/DISABILITY/FACT_SHEET.PHP?SHEET=256 "DISABILITY/CONDITION: SPINA BIFIDA- PHYSICAL ACTIVITY GUIDELINES" ACCESSED ON SEPTEMBER 1, 2011.

5. HTTP://WWW.NCHPAD.COM/DISABILITY/FACT_SHEET.PHP?SHEET=130 "DISABILITY/CONDITION: SPINAL CORD INJURY AND EXERCISE" ACCESSED ON SEPTEMBER 1, 2011.

6. HTTP://WWW.NCHPAD.COM/DISABILITY/FACT_SHEET.PHP?SHEET=62 "DISABILITY/CONDITION: SPINAL CORD INJURY" ACCESSED ON SEPTEMBER 1, 2011.

7. HTTP://WWW.NCHPAD.COM/DISABILITY/FACT_SHEET.PHP?SHEET=63 "DISABILITY/CONDITION: POST POLIOMYELITIS" ACCESSED ON SEPTEMBER 1, 2011.

CHAPTER 18

Non-Progressive Brain Injuries

By Holly Gigure, CTRS, HFS, and Lamont Kelly

Holly Gigure is a Certified Therapeutic Recreation Specialist (CTRS) and ACSM Health Fitness Specialist. She has worked as Courage Center (St. Croix) fitness and aquatic coordinator for 15 years. Holly is trained in Watsu® and aquatic integration and performs aquatic therapy as well as wellness and fitness programming for clients of all abilities and disabilities.

Lamont Kelly has worked as a fitness and aquatic specialist for Courage Center for six years, and works with clients of all abilities and disabilities both in a therapeutic pool and fitness center. Lamont has worked in group homes for many years and is also a certified massage therapist specializing in range of motion and assisted stretching techniques.

Courage Center has been offering comprehensive therapy, sports and recreation, fitness and aquatics, and camping services for people with disabilities for over 80 years.

Stroke

Definition and Cause

A stroke, also called a CVA (cerebrovascular accident), occurs when a blood vessel supplying the brain becomes blocked (ischemic stroke) or when a blood vessel ruptures (hemorrhagic stroke), causing interrupted or reduced blood supply to the brain.[2] This deprives the brain of oxygen and nutrients, which can cause the brain cells to die. Some people may experience a transient ischemic attack (TIA), which is also known as a mini-stroke. Mini-strokes produce a brief period of symptoms similar to those experienced in a stroke, but no permanent damage is sustained. Mini-strokes can be a warning sign for an impending stroke. The National Stroke Association states that "stroke is the third leading cause of death in America and a leading cause of adult disability."[4] Damage from a stroke depends equally on the size and location of the ischemic area.

Table 1 provides known risk factors for stroke.

Symptoms

Symptoms of a stroke can include difficulty walking; difficulty speaking and understanding; confusion; slurred speech; drooling due to loss of tone in facial muscles; diffi-

Table 1. Risk factors for stroke.[6]

Personal or family history of stroke, heart attack or TIA	High cholesterol
High blood pressure	Diabetes
Being age 55 or older	Cardiovascular disease
Sedentary lifestyle	Use of birth control pills or hormone therapies
Smoking or high exposure to second hand smoke	Poor diet
High BMI	Depression

culty finding the right words to explain what is happening; paralysis or numbness on one side of the body or face, sometimes accompanied with a facial droop (side of the face and/or eye); difficulty seeing in one or both eyes; and headache.

Associated and Secondary Conditions

Table 2 provides a list of conditions associated with a stroke.[5] It should be noted that not all stroke survivors will experience all of these conditions.

Table 2. Conditions associated with a stroke.[5]

High and/or low tone in the affected side of the body	Limb and joint pain
Contractures	Depression
Urinary tract infection	Incontinence
Seizures	Circulatory problems within the affected side
Compromised balance	Affected side neglect
Cognitive and communication deficits	Bradykinesia (slow movements)

Comorbidities

Congestive heart failure, diabetes and hypertension are common among stroke survivors. Other comorbidities include recurrent stroke, pulmonary embolism, pneumonia, dyspnea, and major bleeding associated with blood thinners.

Treatment and Medication

Treatment for an ischemic stroke relies on blood flow being quickly returned to the brain. Immediate treatment can improve the likelihood of survival, as well as potentially reducing the complications of the stroke. Medications such as aspirin are used to reduce the likelihood of having another stroke. Doctors sometimes treat ischemic strokes with procedures such as angioplasty and stents. Angioplasty is a technique used to widen the inside of a plaque-coated artery leading to the brain. In this procedure, a balloon-tipped catheter is placed in the blocked area of the artery. The balloon is inflated, squeezing the plaque against the artery walls. A stent is sometimes left in the artery to prevent reoccurring narrowing. Treatment for a hemorrhagic stroke centers on controlling bleeding and reducing pressure in the brain. Surgery may be used to help control future risk.[3]

Exercise Response for Stroke Victims

Certain medications can affect exercise response. It will be important to know if a client is taking blood pressure medication. Expect a client's blood pressure and heart rate to increase while doing cardiovascular exercise, but blood pressure medication should keep levels stationary. Knowing if a client is taking this type of medication is reason to use the rate of perceived exertion (RPE) chart versus using heart rate as a measure of how hard he or she is working. Blood thinners are commonly prescribed for stroke survivors and extra caution should be taken if any type of injury opens the skin. The potential for more serious blood loss is high while taking blood thinners. Also note if the client has a pacemaker. Anti-seizure medications are also sometimes used if clients have had seizures. In addition, it is important to know if the client is susceptible to having seizures and how well the seizures are being managed. Side effects of anti-seizure medications include fatigue, drowsiness, dizziness, double vision, and lack of coordination. Medications like botox and baclofin release muscle tension through chemical interference with the muscle fibers.[1] Be aware that if the dosage is too high, the client can have muscle weakness above and beyond the desired decrease in tone.

Traumatic Brain Injury

Definition and Causes

Traumatic brain injury, also known as TBI, is damage to the brain as the result of an injury. The injury usually results from a violent blow or jolt to the head that causes the brain to collide with the inside of the skull. An object penetrating the skull can also cause traumatic brain injury. A mild TBI may cause temporary dysfunction of brain cells.

Symptoms

Some signs and symptoms of a TBI may appear right away after the traumatic event, while others may appear days or weeks later. The signs and symptoms of a mild traumatic brain injury may consist of: loss of consciousness for a few seconds to a few minutes; no loss of consciousness but a state of being stunned, confused or disoriented; memory or concentration problems; headache; dizziness or loss of balance; nausea or vomiting; sensory problems, such as blurred vision, ringing in the ears or a bad taste in the mouth; sensitivity to light or sound; mood changes or mood swings; feeling depressed or anxious; fatigue or drowsiness, difficulty sleeping or sleeping more than usual. Moderate to severe traumatic brain injury can include any of the signs and symptoms listed above, as well as loss of consciousness from a few minutes to hours, extreme confusion; agitation, combativeness or other unusual behavior; slurred speech; extreme grogginess; weakness or numbness in the extremities; loss of coordination; loss of bladder control or bowel control; persistent headache or headache that worsens; repeated vomiting or nausea; convulsions or seizures; dilation of one or both pupils of the eyes.[11]

Associated and Secondary Conditions

Conditions associated with a stroke are also quite common in a TBI. Depending on the location of the brain injury, one side of the body may be affected, similar to a stroke. See Table 3 for a sampling of conditions connected with TBI, broken into the type of effect. Note that only some of these may happen, depending on the severity and location of the brain injury.

Comorbidities

Clinicians frequently comment that no two traumatic brain injuries are identical. Due to the intricate and often violent nature of their injuries, TBI survivors almost always have numerous acute comorbidities. Most noted is the increased risk for development of severe, long-term psychiatric disorders, particularly major depression, generalized anxiety disorder and post-traumatic stress disorder.[8]

Table 3. Effects of Tramatic Brain Injury.[7]

Physical Effects

Headaches	Communication deficits	Blurry Eyesight
Trouble Hearing	Loss of energy	Affected sense of smell or taste
Dizziness or compromised balance	Contractures	Depression and / or post traumatic stress disorder
High and/or low tone in the affected side of the body	Circulatory problems within the affected side	Seizures
Decreased hand eye coordination	Difficulty swallowing	Vertigo
Limb and joint pain	Affected side neglect	Incontinence

Cognitive Effects

Difficulty concentrating	Forgetfulness	Repeating things
Difficulty making decisions	Difficulty keeping attention and focus	Delayed responses

Behavioral Effects

Easily getting angry	Easily getting frustrated	Acting without thinking
Quick changes in mood	Personality changes	Perseveration

Treatment and Medication

A mild traumatic brain injury may only require rest and over-the-counter pain relievers to treat a headache. However, a person with a mild traumatic brain injury may need monitoring and a follow-up doctor appointment for any persistent, worsening or new symptoms.

Emergency care for moderate to severe traumatic brain injury is centered on making sure the person has a good oxygen and blood supply, stabilizing blood pressure, and preventing any further injury to the head or neck. Medications to limit secondary damage to the brain immediately after an injury may include **diuretics, anti-seizure drugs, and coma-inducing drugs.** Surgery may be needed to reduce further damage to brain tissues, **remove clotted blood (hematomas), repair skull fractures,** and/or to relieve pressure inside the skull.

Medications commonly used for a TBI, include anti-seizure and anti-parkinsonian treatments which are typically used for resting tremors, shuffling gait, swallowing problems, bradykinesia, fatigue, slowed speech, and stimulation/initiation. Other treatments are available for anti-spasticity, antidepressants, antipsychotics, anti-anxiety, and psychostimulants which are helpful for decreased attention/concentration, fatigue, insomnia, and narcolepsy. Common side effects[9] that can impact exercise include:

- anti-seizure–fatigue, drowsiness, dizziness, double vision, lack of coordination
- anti-parkinsonian–dizziness, agitation, low blood pressure, nausea, confusion
- anti-spasticity–drowsiness, weakness, dizziness, nausea, lightheadedness
- antidepressants–headache, nausea, dizziness, agitation, aggressiveness, increased heart rate, drowsiness
- antipsychotics–low blood pressure, seizures, muscle spasms
- anti-anxiety–nausea, drowsiness, dizziness
- psychostimulants–agitation, weight loss, insomnia

Cerebral Palsy

Definition and Causes

Cerebral palsy, also know as CP, is a disorder that is caused by a brain injury occurring before birth, during birthing, or within a few years of birth. The injury (typically anoxic and in utero) affects the brain's ability to control muscles. The effects of this type of TBI may present differently at various stages of a young person's development.

Symptoms

Signs and symptoms of CP appear during infancy or preschool years. Typically, cerebral palsy causes impaired movement problems, such as: differences in muscle tone — either too rigid or too flaccid, stiff muscles and exaggerated reflexes (spasticity), stiff muscles with normal reflexes (rigidity), lack of muscle coordination (ataxia), tremors or involuntary movements, slow movements (bradykinesia), delays in reaching motor skills milestones, favoring one side of the body, and difficulty walking. Some people affected by CP can develop oral dysfunctions such as drooling or difficulty with swallowing, difficulty with sucking or eating, delays in speech development or difficulty speaking. The brain injury causing cerebral palsy doesn't progress, so the symptoms usually don't get worse with age, although the shortening of muscles and muscle rigidity may worsen if not treated.[13]

Associated and Secondary Conditions

People with CP may have other conditions related to developmental brain abnormalities. The disability associated with cerebral palsy may be limited to one limb or one side of the body, or it may affect the entire body. Brain abnormalities as presented in Table 4 are associated with cerebral palsy and may also contribute to other problems.

Table 4. Brain abnormalities associated with Cerebral Palsy.

Intellectual disabilities	Vision and hearing problems	Seizures
Abnormal touch or pain perceptions	dental problems	urinary incontinence
Ataxia and/or athetosis	Altered motor tone	

Treatment and Medication

People with CP will require a continuum of care. The care team may include: a pediatrician or physiatrist, who oversees the treatment plan and medical care; a pediatric neurologist, who specializes in the diagnosis and treatment of neurological disorders in children; an orthopedist, who treats muscle and bone disorders; a physical, occupational, and speech therapist, who assist clients to their highest level of function; a social worker, who assists the family with accessing services and planning for transitions in care; and special education teachers, who address learning disabilities and determine educational needs.

Medications and/or surgeries may be necessary to reduce muscle tension or counteract bone abnormalities caused by chronic spasticity. Certain medications can decrease abnormal tone in muscles and may be used to improve functional abilities, treat pain and manage complications related to spasticity. Baclofen, a muscle relaxer, may be taken orally or be pumped directly into the spinal cord by a surgically implanted pump under the skin of the abdomen. Botox injections may also be used. As mentioned on the section on stroke, these medications can have side effects if dosing is incorrect.

A variety of therapies and alternative services, such as wellness, fitness and aquatic programs can help a person with cerebral palsy to enhance functional abilities. Physical therapy focuses on muscle training and exercises that may help strength, balance, flexibility, motor development and mobility. Braces or splints assist in support and stability and aid in decreasing the development of contractures. Occupational therapy uses alternative strategies and adaptive equipment to promote independent participation in daily activities and routines in the home or community, and/or at school or work. Speech therapy helps improve speech or assists with other forms of communication, such as sign language and/or the use of a Dynavox® product. It may also address difficulties with muscles used in eating and swallowing. Fitness and aquatic specialists can provide additional means for making improvements in a variety of areas. Bodywork modalities such as massage, watsu, and acupuncture can contribute to the overall relaxation and well-being of people with CP.

Developing an Exercise program

Cerebral Palsy (CP), Stroke (CVA) and Traumatic Brain Injury (TBI) have many similarities in regard to exercise testing and programming. As there are varying degrees of severity within each condition, different methods of testing will be appropriate to use. Initially, a physician's approval and description of the client's current condition should be reviewed by the fitness professional. Understanding the aerobic capacity, strength and flexibility of both the affected and non-affected areas will establish a baseline of information that enables the fitness professional to choose an appropriate exercise program. Blood pressure (BP) and heart rate (HR) measurements should be taken throughout the fitness assessment. A Rate of Perceived Exertion (RPE) scale can also assist the fitness professional with getting a comprehensive view of the client's conditioning. Distance and speed travelled may not be an accurate measure of the client's actual level of exertion.

It should be noted that some medications, such as beta blockers, can affect BP/HR. Leg ergometers should be used for aerobic testing with client's who may be unable to stand and/or walk confidently, but are able to maintain their balance while seated and active. Arm/leg ergometers such as the Schwinn® Air-Dyne® and the NuStep® recumbent cross trainers (the T5 NuStep® model has a chest strap accessory available) are options for client's who are able to comfortably incorporate upper extremity movement into the aerobic phase of fitness testing. Treadmills can be used with clients that exhibit the least balance/gait disturbances and lower extremity weakness. For safety, the treadmill should have a minimal start speed (.5 mph or less).

Strength testing options include: Dynamometers which can measure isotonic, isokinetic, and isometric strength, body weight and functional movement exercises (**see examples below**). If possible, the affected limbs should be isolated and tested. When testing an arm or leg, it may be acceptable to avoid hand/wrist and/or ankle articulation in order to get an accurate measure of the range of movement (ROM)/strength of the limb being tested. An example of this would be to use a wrist strap while the client performs a pull down or cable column rear row motion. The muscle group necessary to pulling can be engaged without the limitation of grip strength. For clients with minimal impairments, traditional strength testing options can be used.

Decreased flexibility and ROM are primary issues for clients with any of the three disorders. The fitness professional can establish a baseline for flexibility with the use of a goniometer. Stretching and passive ROM following exercises will provide a thorough "warm-up" period thereby decreasing muscle tension and allowing for a more positive response to stretching.

Some degree of posture and gait will be negatively affected by those with CP, Stroke, or TBI. Controlling one's posture is a function of the somatosensory, visual, and vestibular systems. The client's condition likely has distorted the signals needed to control motion in an efficient and economical manner. Postural changes can be attributed to compensatory changes that provide some degree of balance within the structural limitations of the body. The fitness professional will, through exercise programming, develop a solid foundation from which clients can improve their biomechanics and overall functional movement and balance.

Exercise Programming For Cerebral Palsy, TBI, and Stroke

Traditional standing exercises may need to be performed seated or standing while using a fixed-support structure to ensure safety. Multi-joint/planar exercises are beneficial to develop complex movement retention or muscle memory. An example of this type of exercise would be sit-to-stand exercise. The fitness professional will guide the client through the movement in order to illustrate proper weight distribution and mechanics. During workouts the fitness professional may find that cueing is necessary to ensure consistency throughout exercises. Assisted ROM exercises with a resistive component can incorporate strengthening exercises with a typically passive or unresponsive joint or muscle group. Some exercises allow for strength development of affected areas with the assistance of unaffected muscle groups. In the Figure 1 below, the client's left leg is initiating the movement and hold. The right leg is offering some assistance, however, because the right is crossed over the left, the left side becomes the primary mover. Though this is not a purely unilateral movement, it does illustrate focusing on the affected side actively. This exercise targets the hamstrings and gluteals in an isometric position.

A general fitness plan should follow ACSM guidelines shown in Tables 18.5 and 18.6.[10]

Another option for achieving overall fitness goals involves warm water pool training.

Figure 1.

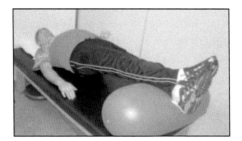

Table 18.5. Stroke and Brain Injury: Exercise Programming

Modes	Goals	Intensity/ Frequency/Duration	Time to Goal
Aerobic • Upper and lower body ergometer • Cycle ergometer • Treadmill • Arm ergometer • Seated stepper	• Increase independence in ADLs • Increase walking speed • Decrease risk of cardio vascular disease	• 40-70% VO_2 peak*; RPE 13/20 • 3-5 days/wk • 20-60 min/session (or multiple 100-min sessions)	2-4 mo
Strength • Isometric exercise • Weight machine • Free weights	• Increase independence in ADLs	• 3 sets of 8-12 reps • 2 days/wk	2-4 mo
Flexibility • Stretching	• Increase ROM of involved extremities • Prevent contractures	• 2 days/wk (before or after Aerobic or • Strength activities)	2-4 mo
Neuromuscular • Coordination and balance activities	• Improve level of safety during ADLs	• 2 days/wk (consider performing on same day as strength activities)	2-4 mo

* VO2 max is undefined in stroke brain injury, and many other neurological pathologies.

Reprinted, with permission, from K. Palmer-McLean and K.B. Harbst, 2003, Stroke and brain injury. In *ACSM's exercise management for persons with chronic diseases and disabilities*, 2nd ed., edited by J.L. Durstine and G.E. Moore for the American College of Sports Medicine (Champaign, IL: Human Kinetics), 243.

Table 18.6. Cerebral Palsy: Exercise Programming

Modes	Goals	Intensity/ Frequency/Duration	Time to Goal
Aerobic • Ambulatory: Schwinn Air Dyne™ Any upper and lower limb ergometer • Wheelchair: Arm ergometer	• Increase aerobic capacity and endurance	• 40-85% VO2 peak or HR reserve • 3-5 days/wk • 20-40 min/session • Emphasize duration over intensity	Variable
Endurance • Ambulatory: 6- to 15-min walks • Wheelchair: 6- to 15-min pushes	• Improve distance covered	• 1-2 sessions/wk	Variable
Strength • Free weights or weight machines	• Improve muscle strength of involved and uninvolved muscle groups	• 3 sets of 8-12 reps • 2 days/wk • Resistance as tolerated	Variable
Flexibility • Stretching (involved and uninvolved joints)	• Improve ROM directly related to capacity for ADls	• Before and after aerobic and endurance exercise	Variable

Reprinted, with permission, from J.J. Laskin, 2003, Cerebral palsy. In *ACSM's exercise management for persons with chronic diseases and disabilities*, 2nd ed., edited by J.L. Durstine and G.E. Moore for the American College of Sports Medicine (Champaign, IL: Human Kinetics), 291.

The warmth of the water offers a near weightless environment allowing the development of functional movement.

Land based functional movement exercises may also be appropriate for clients to improve or maintain activities of daily living skills. Some examples are:

- Sit-to-Stand
- Heel/Toe Walking
- Prone Extension
- Childs Pose
- Ankle Pumps
- Seated Leg Extension
- Rolling

The consistent concerns with all three conditions are excessive tone, spasticity, decreased range of motion and functional movement, decreased cardiovascular/muscular endurance, and loss of flexibility. Over-use injury and affected side neglect are also major concerns. The fitness professional should create an exercise program that addresses all these concerns. Maintaining communication with the client's doctor(s) and family will be important in order to understand the client's current health status and any new precautions that should be taken.

References

1. Gillen, G. and Burkhardt, A., et al. (1998). Stroke Rehabilitation: A Function Based Approach http://www.mayoclinic.org/stroke/ Accessed 13 January 20122012

2. Caplan LR. Etiology and classification of stroke. http://www.uptodate.com/home/index.html. Accessed 7 January 2012.

3. Wiebers, David, M.D. (2001). Stroke Free For Life: The Complete Guide to Stroke Prevention and Treatment. New York, NY. HarperCollins, Inc.

4. National Stroke Association http://www.stroke.org/ Accessed 7 January 2012.

5. Williams CA, Sheppard T, Marrufo M, Galbis-Reig D, Gaskill A, 2003 Jan-Feb;22(1):31-6. A brief descriptive analysis of stroke features in a population of patients from a large urban hospital in Richmond, Virginia, a city within the 'stroke belt'. http://www.ncbi.nlm.nih.gov/pubmed/12566951 Accessed 13 January 2012.

6. Alex Moroz, MD, Ross A. Bogey, DO, Phillip R. Bryant, DO, Carolyn C. Geis, MD, Bryan J. O'Neill, MD, 2004;85(3 Suppl 1):S11-4. Stroke and neurodegenerative disorders. 2. Stroke: comorbidities and complications. http://www.med.nyu.edu/pmr/residency/resources/2-stroke%20comorbidities%20and%20complications.pdf Accessed 14 January 2012.

7. Wilson, Mack. The Effects of Brain Injury on Behavior. http://EzineArticles.com/?expert=Mack_WilsonAccessed 15 January 2012.

8. Rogers JM, Read CA. 2007 Dec;21(13-14):1321-33. Psychiatric comorbidity following traumatic brain injury (abstract).http://www.ncbi.nlm.nih.gov/pubmed/18066935 Accessed 15 January 2012.

9. Winslade, W. (1998). Confronting Traumatic Brain Injury: Devastation, Hope, and Healing. New Haven and London. Yale University Press.

10. Durstine, L. and Moore, G. (2003). ACSM's Exercise Management for Person's with Chronic Diseases and Disabilities, Second Edition. United States of America. Human Kinetics.

11. Braunling-McMorrow D., Niemann G., Savage R. (1998). Training Manual Certified Brain Injury Specialists, Second Edition.

12. Smith,W. (2010). Exercises for Stroke. Hobart, NY. Hatherleigh Press.

13. Miller, F. and Bachrach, S. (2006). Cerebral Palsy: A Complete Guide for Caregiving, Second Edition. Baltimore, Maryland. The Johns Hopkins University Press.

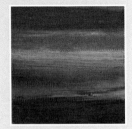

CHAPTER 19

Neuromuscular Conditions

By Kathleen M. Cahill, M.S., RCEP

Kathleen Cahill received her M.S. degree from Northeastern University and B.S. from the University of New Hampshire. Her graduate training in Exercise Science led to a career of clinical exercise physiology positions in Cardiology, Rehabilitation, Research, Health Promotion and faculty positions teaching Clinical Exercise Physiology.

Ms. Cahill is Founder and President of Health Enhancements: medical education solutions, a firm that supports corporations and private practices covering a variety of medical specialties and works with persons with orthopedic and neuromuscular impairments.

She has been a member of ACSM since 1985, serving as CCRB member, ACSM Certification Director and ACSM Workshop Faculty both abroad and in the U.S. She has served on the board of the Clinical Exercise Physiology Association since 2008 and as President (2010-2011). Besides authoring articles and book chapters, Ms. Cahill is also a competitive sailor.

Introduction

Neuromuscular Diseases covered in this chapter are Parkinson's disease, Multiple Sclerosis, Amyotrophic Lateral Sclerosis, Muscular Dystrophy and Fibromyalgia. A consistent practice in working with persons with neuromuscular disorders is to conduct a thorough functional assessment to elucidate the degree of innervation and which muscle groups will need strengthening, stretching, or support during exercise to promote optimal mechanics in gait, posture and exercise performance. Furthermore, emphasis on safety, education, and a multidisciplinary team approach to disease management is essential. The reader should be familiar with exercise guidelines for chronic diseases as established by ACSM and NCHPAD and be able to recognize adverse signs and symptoms or disease progression that may require a consult with the physician and referral to clinical health care providers (*e.g.,* Registered Clinical Exercise Physiologist, occupational therapist, counselor, dietitian).

Parkinson's Disease

Overview of Pathophysiology

Parkinson's Disease (PD) is a progressive, degenerative neurological disorder associated with the loss of dopamine producing cells in the substantia nigra, which is a part of the brain responsible for motor control and voluntary movement. These dopamine pathways control muscle activity but symptoms indicating loss of muscle control do not generally appear until 60-80% of dopaminergic cells have died. The exact cause of PD is unknown, however a combination of genetics, autoimmune deficiencies, injury and environmental exposures to toxins may be contributing factors. The disease usually occurs in individuals over the age of 50.

There are no definitive tests for PD, however, it is classically diagnosed through a neurological exam evaluating the primary symptoms for tremors (at rest or with movement), rigidity (usually begins in neck & shoulders and spreads to trunk & extremities), bradykinesia (decreased ability to move extremities rapidly), and postural instability. Other symptoms include uncontrollable movements (*e.g.,* freezing), muscle cramping, abnormal gait (shuffling and festination), kyphosis (forward rounding of the upper back), difficulty with speech or swallowing, and drooling. The advancing loss of muscle control has secondary effects of muscle atrophy, urinary incontinence, constipation, sensory disorders and skin problems. Resultant comorbidities may include depression, dementia, sleep apnea, vision problems, osteoporosis and erectile dysfunction.[18, 20]

The Hoehn and Yahr scale is commonly used to describe the progression of the disease. The scale is divided into stages from 0 to 5 relative to the level of disability:

Stage 1: Symptoms on one side of the body only. Usually presents with tremor of one limb

Stage 2: Symptoms on both sides of the body, posture and gait affected

Stage 3: Balance impairment, mild to moderate disease, physically independent

Stage 4: Severe disability, but still able to stand or walk unassisted. Rigidity and bradykinesia

Stage 5: Wheelchair bound or bedridden unless assisted

Physiological Considerations and Special Precautions

Autonomic dysfunction from PD can cause abnormal heart rate (HR), blood pressure (BP) and thermal regulation responses. Carefully monitor HR and BP before, during, and after exercise. Control the temperature of the environment (use fans if needed) and encourage proper clothing attire and hydration. Autonomic dysfunction affecting the muscles of the bladder often results in incontinence, and clients will need time to void before and during exercise. If a client has recently undergone Deep Brain Stimulation, (a pacemaker like device implanted in the brain), verify physician clearance for exercise post surgery.[20, 6]

Medications

Some medications have an end of dose 'wear off' time during which the symptoms of PD are exacerbated.

The most common pharmacological agents used to treat PD are Dopaminergics, Peripheral decarboxylase inhibitors, Anticholinergics, Monoamine Oxidase inhibitors, and Catechol-O-methyltransferase inhibitors. Stalevo is the combination of three drugs (levodopa, carbidopa, entacapone) and is currently under review for cardiovascular risk.

There are multiple side effects of the medications such as nausea, arrhythmias, orthostatic hypotension, gastrointestinal irritability, vision, headaches, sleep disturbances, and edema. The potential impact of medications on HR and BP make it important to coordinate the timing of the exercise session around the medication's peak dosage. Moreover, some medications have an end-of-dose 'wear off' time during which the symptoms of PD are exacerbated.[20, 24]

Special Considerations for Exercise Prescription and Programming

A goal for many with PD will be to focus on exercises that improve posture, gait mechanics, and prevent joint contractures or falls. For example, a client with kyphosis will require strength exercises for the back, stretching exercises for chest, hip flexors, and hamstrings, and adjustments to center of gravity while posturing. Muscle rigidity is a

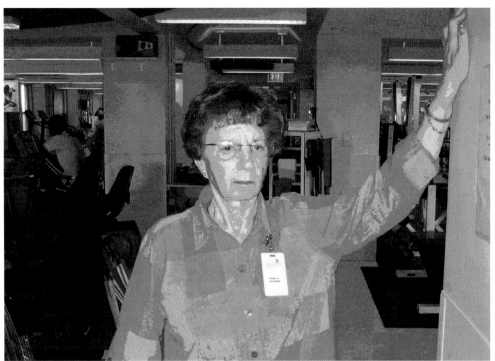

© 2011 National Center on Health, Physical Activity and Disability. Used with permission.

continuous overall increase in muscle tone. In a rigid muscle, resistance is felt with passive range of motion. Early signs of rigidity appear in the trunk and upper extremities. Therefore, exercises focusing on the shoulders and the neck may help maintain function in this area. Some strengthening or flexibility exercises may require active assisted range of motion (ROM) in weakened muscle groups. Muscle spasticity is a sudden increase in muscle tone caused by fast movement through a range of motion. Spasticity can feel intermittent or 'reflexive' because the tightened muscle is resistant to stretch but may not appear with slower movements. Thus the importance of slow, controlled strengthening and flexibility exercises to help reduce spasticity.

Work with your client to establish functional training that will assist with activities of daily living (ADL). Lockette[10, 11] provides numerous examples of exercises to help with ADL functioning such as sit to stand, turning with wide base of support and small steps, and managing stairs. Engage your client in walking as long as they are able but the use of water and recumbent ergometers are also beneficial. Early fatigue is common among persons with PD and may require modification of the duration of exercise (as low as 10 min.) and intensity as tolerated. As Parkinson's progresses and the risk of fall increases, ensure the availability of grab bars, rails, or support devices for all exercises.

Attention to gait correction is an important component of the exercise program. Reinforce principles such as maintaining a wide base of support, take small steps, lift toes before taking a step, avoid movements that require crossing feet, and frequent reminders to swing their arms (if arm swing is diminished).

Another manifestation of PD is freezing (sudden inability to move from disruption of motor control). During exercise, freezing causes a sudden interruption in the activity or makes it difficult to continue. If freezing occurs during an activity, have them stop and refocus on shifting weight from one leg to another, then focus on restarting another move-

May use auditory clues (word/sound) or focus on spot on the floor to get out of a freeze.

ment. Some clients are able to get themselves out of a freeze by using auditory clues (a word or sound) or focusing on a spot on the floor.

A client with frequent freezing, advanced gait problems, severe spasticity, contractures (shortened muscle due to prolonged muscle spasticity around a joint) and bradykinesia may require referral to a clinical professional. As with many neuromuscular diseases, support groups, proper nutrition, and adjunct treatments such as therapeutic massage, acupuncture, or water therapy are encouraged.[10, 11]

Multiple Sclerosis (MS)

Overview of Pathophysiology

Multiple Sclerosis (MS) is a degenerative inflammatory disease of the central nervous system (CNS) where the myelin sheath around the nerve is slowly destroyed, leaving lesions or sclerosis. MS is diagnosed through neurological testing, lab work and magnetic resonance imaging. The clinical course of MS follows a number of patterns ranging from varying lengths of remission/relapse/exacerbation to a slow, progressive decline without any periods of remission. A definitive cause is unknown however specific genes have now been identified that increase one's susceptibility to MS and viral exposure has been postulated as a cause.

The demyelination in multiple areas impairs nerve conduction resulting in symptoms of severe fatigue, 'pins and needles' sensations, pain, tremors, weakness in the extremities, impaired balance, muscle spasticity and paralysis. Secondary conditions include depression, hearing loss, difficulty with concentration and memory, urinary incontinence, high incidence of UTIs, and severe constipation.[8, 5]

Physiological Considerations and Special Precautions

Autonomic nervous system dysfunction, as a result of MS, can affect thermoregulation, HR and diminish BP responses to exercise.

Monitor the following:

- HR and BP before, during, and after exercise.
- Control environment (cool room temperature, low humidity and utilize fans if needed).
- Encourage proper hydration, and clothing attire.
- Maintain adequately cool pool temperatures for water exercises.

Blurred vision during exercise may be caused by optic neuritis (inflammation of the optic nerve) and physician referral is needed.[8,18] Consider clients who will need time to void before and during the session if they have urinary dysfunction (a common feature of MS).

Medications

Various medications are used to manage the symptoms of MS but undesirable side effects complicate disease management. Prophylactic treatments for MS include the use of glatiramer, chemotherapy agents and interferon (avonex, rebif, betaseron) which may produce flu-like symptoms or injection site irritation. Exacerbation periods are treated with high doses of steroids (prednisone, solumedrol) but prolonged use of these agents may cause muscle weakness, fatigue, hypertension, diabetes, osteoporosis or reduced ability to sweat. Other medications used to treat associated symptoms for urinary dysfunction, constipation and spasms may also cause muscle weakness and fatigue. Ampyra (dalfampridine) was approved in 2010 for the improvement of walking in patients with MS.[24]

Special Considerations for Exercise Prescription and Programming

The goal for persons with MS is to maintain cardiovascular health, strength, flexibility, balance and manage spasticity. The general guidelines for prescribing activity for persons with MS as noted by ACSM and NCHPAD are appropriate for most clients. However, a thorough functional assessment will provide maximal benefits in maintaining good mechanics and posture. During the initial stages of MS, when lower extremity impairments are minimal, increasing leg strength will result in better walking performance (avoid treadmill walking if foot drop is present). Water exercises (temp. 81-84 degrees), yoga, recumbent cycle ergometers and arm ergometers are the mode of choice when balance and spasticity become problematic. Although resistance training is beneficial, avoid strengthening hypertrophied muscles and do not use free weights if your client develops sensory deficits.

Gait characteristics of those with advancing spasticity and muscle weakness exhibit ankle supination, pronation, inversion and eversion, leg valgus and varus, scissor gait, hip circumduction and compensatory arm swing. For tight muscle groups around the ankle, knee and hip, gently hold stretches for 1-2 minutes. When mild spasticity is present, strengthen the opposing muscle group. Spastic muscle groups that are incapable of being strengthened due to ROM limitations should be gently stretched. For example, a person whose gait exhibits "toe walking" should be taught to slowly stretch the gastrocnemius of the affected side. However, do not stretch a muscle in acute spasm and consult a physician or clinical provider if severe spasticity exists.

During early stages, increase leg strength to improve walking.

Fatigue is a very common symptom in those with MS and can be disabling. Morning exercise sessions are usually the best time for clients before weariness of the day sets in. Include the use of the fatigue scale and if extreme fatigue exists post exercise, modify the exercise prescription (intensity, duration) to tolerance. Likewise, the exercise regimen will need to be adjusted during periods of exacerbation and remission with possible use of adaptive devices to hold weights (mitt or glove) or straps to keep hands and feet on ergometers. Overall, choose modes where risk of falling is minimized.[8, 15, 16]

Amyotrophic Lateral Sclerosis

Overview of Pathophysiology

Amyotrophic Lateral Sclerosis (ALS or "Lou Gehrig's") is an idiopathic progressive degeneration of the upper and lower motor neurons in the CNS with only a small percentage who have inherited a genetic mutation. Amyotrophic refers to muscle atrophy and sclerosis refers to the scar tissue created along the nerves. ALS accounts for 10 percent of all adult onset motor neuron disease. In most cases the progression of ALS is rapid (survival rate 5 yrs.) and ultimately leads to respiratory failure. The cause of ALS is unknown and is diagnosed with symptoms of upper and lower motor neuron damage in the medulla (bulbar or oropharyngeal), cervical, thoracic, and lumbar regions.

Classic ALS involves both the upper and lower motor neurons resulting in muscle weakness, spasticity, uncontrolled movements, cognitive impairment, and oropharyngeal degeneration (problems with swallowing, slurred speech, and drooling).[21]

Physiological Considerations and Special Precautions

*Monitor;
Joint laxity
Injury
Pulmonary
function*

Because ALS is progressive and functional ability decreases despite any amount of exercise, the goal of the exercise program is to keep them active for as long as possible. Special precaution should be taken regarding joint laxity, injury due to denervated limbs, and decreased pulmonary function as respiratory muscles fail with disease progression. Comorbidities include depression and anxiety.[3]

Medications

One drug that has been approved for the treatment of ALS and has been shown to prolong survival (slightly) by inhibiting glutamate release, is Riluzol (rilutec). All other medications are administered to treat symptoms (spasticity, depression, swallowing, etc). The side effects of fatigue and muscle weakness from these drugs may require modification of the exercise program as tolerated. The medications to control side effects may include: (1) Nuedexta for uncontrolled expression of emotion or the 'pseudobulbar effect'; (2) an investigational insulin growth factor; (3) Myotrophin to help decrease spasticity and uncontrolled movements; and (4) antidepressants.[21]

Special Considerations for Exercise Prescription and

Programming

The main goals in the early stages of ALS are to preserve strength, prevent muscle atrophy of the functioning innervated areas, and prevent contractures through ROM and stretching. In the early stage, the order of ROM exercises is active ROM first, then active assistive followed by passive ROM. Avoid excessive repetition and high intensity activities at all times. As there are no remissions with ALS, impairments will only continue to increase and ability to perform exercises will decrease. It is important that the patient and health professional understand this and set goals accordingly. Adaptive devices for equipment may be needed as functional ability decreases.

Psychosocial and nutritional support are important components to a well rounded program. The progressing disease severely affects gait, balance, ADL, range of motion, spasticity along with contractures and will require referral to a clinical professional.[3]

Muscular Dystrophy

Overview of Pathophysiology

Muscular Dystrophy (MD) is a group of more than 30 genetic degenerative muscle diseases resulting in muscle cell death in both children and adults. The rate of progression and extent of muscle dysfunction varies among the various forms of MD. Some of the more common types are presented in Table 1.

The symptoms vary depending on the type of MD but include muscle weakness, atrophy, abnormal gait, joint contractures, drooling, drooping eyelids, impaired speech, and

Table 1: Common Types of Muscular Dystrophy

Type	Cause	Muscular Dysfunction
Duchenne (DMD)	defective gene for a protein called dystrophin	rapid decline & begins proximally in the legs and pelvis and spreads distally to the arms, trunk, and neck
Becker	insufficient production of the dystrophin protein	like Duchenne's but progresses more slowly
Emery-Dreifuss	defective gene that produces proteins in the sarcolemma	slowly progresses primarily in skeletal muscles, ultimately affecting the cardiac muscle
Facioscapulohumeral (FSMD)	missing piece of DNA, teenage onset	slow progression, affecting muscles of the face, shoulder, upper arms and chest
Limb-girdle	defective gene that affects muscle proteins	slowly progresses in shoulders and hips
Distal Muscular	defective muscle protein	hands, forearms, and lower legs
Myotonic Dystrophy	defect on the DNA causing muscle wasting and inability of muscles to relax, teen or adult onset (Myotonic Congenita is a more severe form, appears at birth)	face, neck, arms, legs

prolonged muscle spasms. Clients may also experience problems with cataracts, osteoarthritis, osteoporosis, skeletal deformities (e.g., scoliosis), thermoregulation, cardiomyopathy, arrhythmias (conduction blocks), CHF, pneumonia, and respiratory failure. Cognitive impairment varies and is not seen in all types.[22, 18]

Physiological Considerations and Special Precautions

Arrhythmias, shortness of breath and temperature regulation should be monitored carefully. Due to potential cardiovascular compromise, a Certified Inclusive Fitness Trainer (CIFT) should obtain exercise test results and physician clearance before beginning an exercise program. Special precaution should be taken to maintain a temperate environment (avoid high heat/humidity and cold for those with myotonic dystrophies).

Medications

Medications are prescribed for the symptoms of MD as there are no medications that treat the cause. Steroids can result in weight gain, hypertension, hyper/hypoglycemia, muscle weakness joint laxity, and decreased tolerance to activity. Long term steroid use can also cause hyperlipidemia, cataracts, and osteoporosis. Beta-2 agonists may be prescribed for FSMD and can cause arrhythmias. Other medications commonly used for MD include acetaminophen, non-steriodal anti-inflammatories, immunosuppressive agents (methotrexate, and azathioprine), creatine monohydrate (possibly increase exercise capacity) and anti spasmodic or muscle relaxants (diazepam, baclofen, dantrolene sodium). For CIFTs working with children as part of a multidisciplinary team, Bushby[4] provides detailed information on the complications and management of Duchenne's in children.

Special Considerations for Exercise Prescription and Programming

Resistance training; Water Exercise bands Manual resistance

ACSM provides appropriate guidelines for exercise prescription on those with muscular dystrophies. For those with MD, the goal is to preserve strength and perform gentle stretching or ROM to help prevent contractures. Evaluation of posture, gait, balance, strength, and flexibility will provide the foundations to the exercise prescription. In order to maintain the ability to perform ADL, encourage walking and standing for as long as they are able to do so. Most clients will need a long, slow warm up and cool down with prolonged stretching periods and modified intensity and duration of aerobic activity due to early fatigue. Water and the use of exercise bands in the antigravity position are excellent modes for resistance training (free weights are not recommended). Allow 48 hrs of rest between muscle strengthening sessions for a given muscle group. Providing passive ROM, active assistive ROM, or minimal manual resistance in the antigravity position may be necessary in the case of extremely tight or weakened muscle groups.

Contraindications to exercise include muscle cramping, discolored urine, prolonged muscle pain (>48 hrs) or progressive loss of strength (refer to the physician or a clinical professional). Strength exercises are contraindicated in myotonic dystrophies due to extreme muscle hypertrophy and inability of muscles to relax. If respiratory function begins to decline, referral to the physician and a clinician for inspiratory muscle training is indicated.[12, 22]

Fibromyalgia

Overview of Pathophysiology

Fibromyalgia (FM) is a syndrome of unknown etiology and characterized by widespread chronic pain. A disruption of the autonomic nervous system causes sensory processing pathways to be in a state of disarray. It affects more women than men and is diagnosed by the results of a physical exam and the American College of Rheumatology (ACR) criteria which focuses on multiple tender points and self-reported symptoms. In some cases, identification of certain triggers such as a life altering event or recent trauma have been related to the onset of FM.

Symptoms include diffuse musculoskeletal pain, with various areas that are tender to the touch (tender points), deep aching, stabbing or shooting pain, numbness, tingling, twitching, headaches and extreme fatigue. As one can imagine, being in a state of chronic pain results in a myriad of problems with sleep, vision (sensitivity to light), skin (sensitivity to touch), auditory (tinitus, dizziness), stress, anxiety, depression, trouble concentrating and further fatigue. Many with FM also experience autoimmune conditions such as lupus, arthritis, and irritable bowel.

*http://www.
rhuematology.org/
practice/clinical*

Physiological Considerations and Special Precautions

The disrupted autonomic nervous system may cause problems with thermoregulation, HR and blunted BP response to exercise. Triggers that exacerbate symptoms include (but are not limited to) cold and humid environment, excessive physical activity as well as inactivity, anxiety and stress. Chronic fatigue and pain symptoms are very daunting for the CIFT and client. Therefore, it is extremely important to work closely with the client in establishing achievable goals and collaborate with a multidisciplinary team.

Medications

As a result of dopamine depletion from an overactive sympathetic system in FM, the most common medications for pain management are dopamine agonists. These include pregabalin (Lyrica), duloxetine (Cymbalta) and milnacipran (Savella) which are unlikely to have an effect on the exercise response. However, other medications used to treat secondary symptoms or comorbid conditions may have an adverse affect on the exercise response. Obtain this list of medications to determine adverse side effects or negative impact upon the exercise response.[1, 9]

Special Considerations for Exercise Prescription and Programming

Although exercise itself can result in fatigue, pain and frustration for FM clients, the deleterious effects of inactivity are unfavorable. The main goal of the exercise program is to provide enjoyable, low level activities and gentle stretching that will help maintain (or restore) functional levels. Advance your client *very* slowly beginning with short duration (possibly as low as 10-15 min.), low intensity (40-50% HRR), 2 days per week at a time of day that is least symptomatic for the client. Cycling, yoga, tai chi, water aerobics and swimming are modes of choice for low impact activities. Exercises performed in a warm therapeutic pool (93-96 degrees) may provide relief from pain but if thermoregulatory control is compromised, limit time in the pool and monitor HR and BP carefully. Recumbent bicycles may be better tolerated than standard bicycle ergometers for those with gluteal tenderpoints. Avoid the following: (1) high impact or high intensity exercise; (2) eccentric contractions; (3) sustained overhead exercises; and (4) morning exercise sessions (due to stiffness and fatigue from lack of sleep).

Most importantly, incorporate other components into your client's program such as relaxation techniques (*e.g.*, deep breathing, mental imagery), proper nutrition, support groups and healthy sleep routines (*i.e.*, avoid caffeine, alcohol, noise, computer and television viewing distractions before bed, practice relaxation techniques lying in bed). Alternative treatments may also include acupuncture, osteopathic manipulation, tai chi, aromatherapy, cryotherapy and therapeutic heat.[7, 9, 17, 19]

Summary

Many neuromuscular disorders are complex. The varying level of impairment, progression rates, direct effects, indirect effects, or client's level of motivation can make such conditions challenging to manage for the professional. For example, muscular weakness can be a direct result of the disease or an indirect effect of medication or disuse. It is important the CIFT recognize that each neuromuscular disease state is unique and modifications must be tailored to maximize the functional ability of each client.

References

1. ACSM's Guidelines for Exercise Testing and Prescription, 8th ed. Baltimore: Lippincott Williams & Wilkins, 2010

2. Arnold, L. M., Clauw, D. J., & McCarberg, B. H. (2011). Improving the Recognition and Diagnosis of Fibromyalgia. Mayo Clinic Proceedings, 86(5), 457-464. doi:10.4065/mcp.2010.0738

3. Bello-Haas, V.D. & Krivickas, L. S. (2009). Amyotrophic Lateral Sclerosis. In J. Durstine, G. Moore, P. Painter & S. Roberts (Eds.), ACSM's exercise management for persons with chronic diseases and disabilities (3rd ed., pp. 336-342). Champaign, IL: Human Kinetics.

4. Bushby, K., Bourke, J., Bullock, R., Eagle, M., Gibson, M. & Quinby, J. (2005). The multidisciplinary management of duchenne muscular dystrophy. Current Paediatrics, 15, 292-300. doi:10.1016/j.cupe.2005.04.001

5. Carroll, C.C. & Lambert, C.P. (2009). Multiple Sclerosis. In J. Ehrman, P. Gordon, P. Visich & S. Keteyian (Eds.), Clinical exercise physiology (2nd ed.) Champaign, IL: Human Kinetics.

6. Goodwin VA, Richards SH, Taylor RS, Taylor AH, Campbell JL. The effectiveness of exercise interventions for people with Parkinson's disease: a systematic review and meta-analysis. Mov Disord. 2008 Apr 15;23(5):631-40.

7. Gowans, S.E. & deHueck, A. (2004). Effectiveness of exercise in management of fibromyalgia: effect of exercise on physical function. Current Opinion in Rheumatology 16(2) © 2004 Lippincott Williams & Wilkins. http://www.medscape.com/viewarticle/470554_2

8. Jackson, K. & Mulcare, J. (2009). Multiple Sclerosis. In J. Durstine, G. Moore, P. Painter & S. Roberts (Eds.), ACSM's exercise management for persons with chronic diseases and disabilities (3rd ed., pp. 321-326). Champaign, IL: Human Kinetics.

9. Lemley, K & Meyer, B. (2009). Fibromyalgia. In J. Durstine, G. Moore, P. Painter & S. Roberts (Eds.), ACSM's exercise management for persons with chronic diseases and disabilities (3rd ed., pp. 239-245). Champaign, IL: Human Kinetics

10. Lockette, K. (2009). Move It: An exercise and movemement guide for people with parkinson's disease. Minneapolis, MN: Langdon Street Press. ISBN 1934938297

11. Lockette, K. & Keyes, A. (1994). Conditioning with physical disabilities. Champaign, IL: Human Kinetics.

12. Markert, C.D., Ambrosio, F., Call, J.A., Grange, R.W. (2011). Exercise and duchenne muscular dystrophy: toward evidence-based exercise prescription. Muscle Nerve 43:(4), 464-478. doi:10.1002/mus.21987 PMID:21404285

13. Morin, A. K. (2009). Fibromyalgia: A review of management options. Formulary, 44(12), 362.

14. Muscular Dystrophy Association. http://www.mda.org

15. National Center on Health, Physical Activity and Disability. www.nchpad.org/disability

16. National Multiple Sclerosis Society. www.nmss.org

17. NIH National Institute of Arthritis and Mucsuloskeletal and Skin Diseases. www.niams.nih.gov

18. NIH National Institute of Neurological Disorders and Stroke (NINDS) . www.ninds.nih.gov/disorders/disorder_index.htm

19. Ortega, E. E., Bote, M. E., Giraldo, E. E., & García, J. J. (2012). Aquatic exercise improves the monocyte pro- and anti-inflammatory cytokine production balance in fibromyalgia patients. Scandinavian Journal Of Medicine & Science In Sports, 22(1), 104-112. doi:10.1111/j.1600-0838.2010.01132.x

20. Protas, E.J., Stanley, E.K., & Jankovic, J. (2009). Parkinson's disease. In J. Durstine, G. Moore, P. Painter & S. Roberts (Eds.), ACSM's exercise management for persons with chronic diseases and disabilities (3rd ed., pp. 350-356). Champaign, IL: Human Kinetics.

21. Rowland, L.P. & Shneider, N.A. (2001). Amyotrophic lateral sclerosis New England Journal of Medicine, 344(22), 1688-1700. Retrieved from http://www.nejm.org

22. Tarnopolsky, M.A. (2009). Muscular Dystrophy. In J. Durstine, G. Moore, P. Painter & S. Roberts (Eds.), ACSM's exercise management for persons with chronic diseases and disabilities (3rd ed., pp. 306-312). Champaign, IL: Human Kinetics

23. Traynor, L. M., Thiessen, C. N., & Traynor, A. P. (2011). Pharmacotherapy of fibromyalgia. American Journal Of Health-System Pharmacy, 68(14), 1307-1319. doi:10.2146/ajhp100322

24. U.S. Food and Drug Administration. http://www.fda.gov. http://www.fda.gov/Drugs/DrugSafety/ucm223060.htm

25. Wolfe F., Smythe HA, Yunus MB et al. The American College of Rheumatology 1990 criteria for the classification of fibromyalgia. Arthritis Rheumatology. 1990;33:160-72. retrieved Jan. 21,2012 from http://www.rheumatology.org/practice/clinical/classification/fibromyalgia/2010_Preliminary_Diagnostic_criteria.pdf]

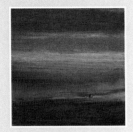

CHAPTER 20

Cognitive Disabilities

By Donna Bernhardt Bainbridge, PT, Ed.D., ATC

Donna Bainbridge received her professional education and doctoral degree at Boston University, and her master's degree at the University of North Carolina. Currently Special Olympics Senior Global Advisor for FUNfitness and Fitness Programming, she is directing the development and assessment of fitness screening and programming for athletes around the globe. She is also Adjunct Faculty at the University of Indianapolis, teaching Health Promotion and Wellness. She works in the Physical Therapy Clinic at the University of Montana, and is a Consultant in Wellness programs for people with intellectual disabilities at the University of Montana Rural Institute.

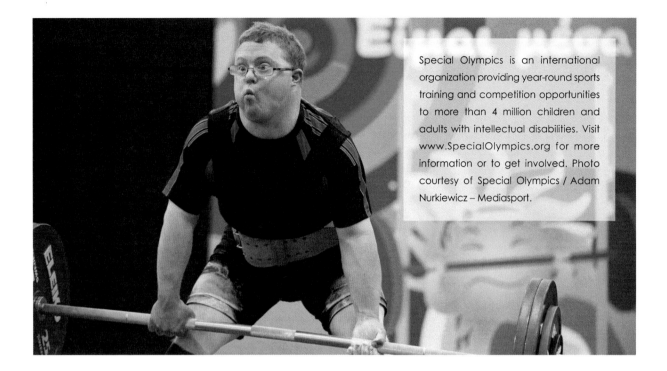

Special Olympics is an international organization providing year-round sports training and competition opportunities to more than 4 million children and adults with intellectual disabilities. Visit www.SpecialOlympics.org for more information or to get involved. Photo courtesy of Special Olympics / Adam Nurkiewicz – Mediasport.

PART I
INTELLECTUAL DISABILITY

Overview of the Condition

A person with an intellectual disability, as defined by the American Association on Intellectual and Development Disability,[1] is an individual with significant limitations in both intellectual functioning and adaptive behavior (conceptual, social and practical skills). Intellectual functioning is usually measured with an IQ test; an IQ score of 70 or less indicates a limitation in intellectual functioning. Standardized tests can also determine limitations in adaptive behavior.

Intellectual disability (ID) is a subset within the larger category of developmental disability. Developmental disabilities (DD) are defined as chronic disabilities that can be cognitive, physical or both. Some DD, such as congenital deafness, are totally physical. Other DD, including cerebral palsy or spina bifida, may or may not include ID. Yet others, such as Down, fetal alcohol, and Fragile X Syndrome are frequently associated with ID. Both developmental and intellectual disabilities appear before the age of 18 and are present for life.

The term previously applied to people with ID was mental retardation. The change of term to *intellectual disability* emphasizes that ID is not an invariable trait of a person, and opens the way to self-worth, pride, community engagement and employment. The term 'intellectual disability' also has less negative and offensive connotation.[41]

As many as 3 of every 100 people (3%) in this country have an intellectual disability.[8,9]

In 2004, special education and related services were being received by 6,118,437 students ages six through 21 which represents 9.2 % of the U.S. general population of these ages. Nine percent of children who need special education have some form of ID, and one in 10 families is affected by ID.[47]

Approximately 85% of the ID population is in the mild category (IQ from 50 to 75); they can acquire academic skills, become fairly self-sufficient, and live independently with community and social support. About 10% of the ID population is in the moderate group with IQ scores from 35 to 55. They can carry out self-care and work tasks with supervision, and are able to live successfully within a supervised community environment. Only 3% to 4% of the population has severe ID (IQ scores of 20 to 40), yet they can master basic self-care and communication skills, and many are able to live in a group environment. The remaining 1% to 2% is classified as profoundly involved with IQ scores under 20 to 25. They may be able to develop basic self-care and communication skills with appropriate support and training, but usually need a high level of structure and supervision. Hence, every person with intellectual disability is able to learn, develop, and grow, and live a satisfying life.[5]

Approximately 40% to 50% of the cases of intellectual disabilities have no identifiable origin.[7] However, the most common general causal categories are:

- *Genetic conditions:* Sometimes ID is caused by problems with genes: abnormal genes inherited from parents or errors when genes combine. Examples are Down syndrome, Fragile X Syndrome, and phenylketonuria (PKU).

- *Problems during pregnancy:* ID can result when the baby does not develop properly in-utero. For example, there may be a problem with the way the baby's cells divide as it grows. A woman who gets an infection like rubella during pregnancy or ingests alcohol may have a baby with ID.[22,45]

- *Problems at birth:* If a baby has problems during labor and delivery (*i.e.,* not getting enough oxygen, or having the umbilical cord wrapped around the neck) he or she may have an ID.

- *Health or societal problems:* Diseases like whooping cough, measles, or meningitis can cause ID. ID can also be caused by extreme malnutrition, poor medical care, or exposure to poison like lead or mercury. ID can also be caused by social factors, such as stimulation level, and educational factors, such as the availability of family and educational supports that promote mental development and adaptive skills.[25,51]

There are hundreds of syndromes and conditions that can be associated with ID. Each of these syndromes may be associated with one or more primary complications, such as cognitive or sensory impairment, seizures, neuro-motor dysfunction, and syndrome-specific conditions such as cardiac defects or other physical malformations. Any primary complication may lead to secondary health consequences, known as secondary conditions.

These can include obesity, osteoporosis, or diabetes to name a few.

Several types of ID are more commonly encountered in the United States.

Down syndrome

Down syndrome, the most frequently occurring chromosomal disorder, occurs in approximately one in every 800 live births, and accounts for 15% of all cases of ID.[17] Individuals with Down syndrome have 47 instead of the usual 46 chromosomes. It is usually caused by an error in cell division that occurs at conception and is not related to anything done during pregnancy. The incidence of Down syndrome increases with advancing maternal age; however, 80% of children with Down syndrome are born to women under 35 years of age. Down syndrome is not related to race, nationality, religion or socioeconomic status.

Down syndrome is usually identified at or shortly after birth. The initial diagnosis is based on physical characteristics commonly seen in babies, including low muscle tone, a single crease across the palm, a slightly flattened facial profile and an upward slant to the eyes. The diagnosis must be confirmed by a chromosome study.

Children with Down syndrome experience delays in physical and intellectual development. Most children attend school, some in regular and others in special education classes. Some high school graduates with Down syndrome participate in post-secondary education, and many adults with Down syndrome are capable of working in the community, some requiring a more structured.[30]

Many children with Down syndrome have additional health complications.[39] Approximately 40% have congenital heart defects, so an echocardiogram should be performed on all newborns with Down syndrome to identify the presence of any serious cardiac problems. Some of these heart conditions require surgery while others only need monitoring.[11,16,26] Children with Down syndrome have a higher incidence of respiratory, vision and hearing problems, thyroid and other metabolic conditions, and sleep disturbances including sleep apnea. Atlanto-axial instability (AAI) can be observed by x-ray in 15% of people with Down syndrome, but in about 90% of these cases (13%–14% of people with Down syndrome) the AAI is asymptomatic. A link between spinal cord injury and AAI exists in only 1% of people with Down syndrome who are.[2,4,19]

With appropriate medical care most individuals with Down syndrome lead healthy lives. Average life expectancy is 55 years, with many living into their sixties and seventies. People with Down syndrome may experience similar health problems as they age to those experienced by all older people. However, the presence of the extra genetic material and the fact that they age prematurely (*i.e.,* show physical changes related to aging 20 to 30 years ahead of people of the same age in the general population) may lead to abnormalities in the immune system and a higher susceptibility to certain illnesses, such as leukemia, seizures, cataracts, breathing problems, and heart conditions.

Individuals over 40 with Down syndrome who have a family member with Alzheimer disease are at greater risk of developing Alzheimer disease. The hallmark lesions of Alzheimer disease are present in the brains of all adults with Down syndrome by the age 40, which suggests a shared genetic susceptibility to both conditions.[13] Although the characteristic tangles and plaques do not mean that all individuals with Down syndrome will develop Alzheimer disease, it is well documented that the prevalence of dementia increases with age in persons with Down syndrome. Adults with Down syndrome often are in their mid to late 40s or early 50s when Alzheimer symptoms first appear. Studies estimate that clinical and behavioral symptoms of Alzheimer disease will be present in approximately 50%–70% of individuals with Down syndrome by the time they reach 60 years.[50,30]

The symptoms and progression of Alzheimer disease in the Down syndrome population present somewhat differently. The progression of Alzheimer disease for persons with Down syndrome takes about eight years. Symptoms are sometimes subtle and difficult to define because of the pre-existing cognitive impairments. Some of these symptoms may include: personality changes, loss of speech or change in language skills, disorientation to time and place, decline in self-care skills, abrupt onset of new seizure activity, incontinence in an individual who has always been independent, development or increase of short-term memory loss, and disruptions in sleep-wake cycles.[23,36]

Fragile X Syndrome

Fragile X Syndrome (FXS), the most common cause of inherited mental impairment, is a genetic condition caused by a change in the FMR1 gene on the X chromosome. The change in the gene, which is responsible for making a protein that is important in brain development, causes it to work improperly. (See Table 20.1). Consequently, brain function including learning, behavior and communication is affected. Approximately 1 in 3,600 to 4,000 males worldwide is born with full mutation for Fragile X (37,179 in U.S.); the vast majority of males with this full mutation will have FXS. Approximately 1 in

Table 20.1[32]

Physical Features (males and some females, except where noted)	Behavioral, Intellectual, and Social Characteristics	Difficulties for Adults	Issues Common in Females including some carriers	Important Family History Questions
• Large/protruding ears • Recurrent otitis media in child • Soft skin • Flexible joints (particularly fingers, wrists, elbows) • Low muscle tone • Flat feet • Long face • Large testicles • Seizure disorder	• Speech and language delay • Motor delay. • Tactile defensiveness and sensory overload. • Hand-flapping, hand-biting • Impulsivity • Poor eye contact/gaze aversion • Autism spectrum disorders-ADHD, • Cognitive impairment or ID	• Managing transitions. • Learning adult living skills such as using transportation and money • Managing emotional upsets without aggressive behavior • Making and sustaining friendships	• Visual-spatial challenges like reading maps and graphs. • Executive functioning (ability to form, execute, and follow a plan) • Mathematics • Shyness or social anxiety • Poor communication skills • Difficulty in picking up "social cues" • Anxiety, mood swings and depression	• Family history of learning disabilities, mental impairment, including autism and other behavioral disorders. • Family history of female relatives with infertility, early or premature menopause • Family history of adults (particularly men) with late (after 50) onset neurological findings including intention tremor, ataxia, memory or cognitive decline, personality or psychiatric changes

National Fragile X Foundation, 2010

4,000 to 6,000 females worldwide (approximately 38,400 in U.S.) are born with full mutation for Fragile X, but only 50% of females with this full mutation will have some features of FXS.   FXS is the most common *known* cause of autism or "autistic-like" behaviors.[28] Symptoms also can include characteristic physical and behavioral features and delays in speech and language development.[40]

Prader-Willi

Prader-Willi syndrome (PWS) is the most common genetic cause of life-threatening obesity in children, resulting from an abnormality on the 15th chromosome. It occurs equally in males and females and in all races. Prevalence estimates range from 1:8,000 to 1:25,000 (most likely 1:15,000). PWS affects approximately 1 in 10,000 to 1 in 25,000 newborns.[16] The infant typically has low birth weight, low muscle tone with difficulty sucking, which can lead to a diagnosis of failure to thrive. The second stage of 'thriving too well' has a typical onset at two and five years. Children with PWS have loving personalities, but also increased appetite, weight control issues, speech and motor development delays along with behavior problems and unique medical issues. PWS typically causes low muscle tone, short stature if not treated with growth hormone, incomplete sexual development, and a chronic feeling of hunger that, coupled with a metabolism that utilizes drastically fewer calories than normal, can lead to excessive eating and life-threatening obesity.[18,38] The food compulsion makes constant supervision necessary.[34]

Their extreme unsatisfied drive to consume food lasts a lifetime.[27] Adults are often infertile, obese, and prone to diabetes. They are hypotonic and extremely flexible. General appearance includes a prominent nasal bridge, almond-shaped eyes with thin, downturned lids, and high narrow forehead. They have excess abdominal fat and soft skin that is easily bruised Average IQ is 70, but even those with normal IQs have learning issues. Social and motor deficits also exist.[43]

They are often strong in visual organization and perception, but spoken language is generally poorer than comprehension. Auditory information and sequential processing are poor, as are arithmetic and writing skills, visual and auditory short term memory and auditory attention span. These sometimes improve with age.

The main mental health difficulties experienced by people with PWS include compulsive behavior (manifested in skin-picking) and anxiety.[3] Psychiatric symptoms affect approximately 5%–10% of young adults.

Autism Spectrum Disorders

Autism is a complex neuro-developmental disorder defined by qualitative impairments in communication and social interactions, restricted interests and activities, and stereotypical behaviors. All individuals have qualitative abnormalities of social development with disorders of communication and/or stereotyped repetitive interests and behaviors. Natural social skills do not develop; as children mature, these characteristics can change but the diagnosis remains.[29, 43]

Symptoms usually start before age three, and can cause delays or problems in many skills that develop from infancy to adulthood. Different people with autism can have very different symptoms. Autism is a "spectrum," a group of disorders with similar features. Currently, the autism spectrum disorder (ASD) category includes: autistic disorder ("classic" autism), Asperger syndrome, and Pervasive Developmental Disorder Not Otherwise Specified (or atypical autism). The main signs and symptoms of autism involve problems in the following areas:[30, 31]

- Communication: both verbal and non-verbal (*i.e.,* pointing, eye contact, and smiling)
- Social: sharing emotions, understanding how others think/feel, and having a conversation
- Routines or repetitive behaviors such as repeating words or actions, obsessively following routines or schedules, and playing in repetitive ways.

There are many possible behaviors that may be signs or symptoms for autism. For example, the child:

- does not respond to his/her name.
- cannot explain what he/she wants.
- may be slow to develop speech or language skills.
- doesn't follow directions.
- at times, seems to be deaf.
- seems to hear sometimes, but not other times.
- doesn't point or wave "bye-bye."
- used to say a few words or babble, but now he/she doesn't.
- throws intense or violent tantrums.
- has odd movement patterns.
- is overly active, uncooperative, or resistant.
- doesn't know how to play with toys.
- doesn't smile when smiled at.
- has poor eye contact.
- gets stuck doing the same things repeatedly and can't move to other things.
- seems to prefer to play alone.
- gets things for him/herself only.
- is very independent for his/her age.
- does things "early" compared to other children.
- seems to be in his/her "own world."
- seems to tune people out.
- is not interested in other children.
- walks on his/her toes.
- shows unusual attachments to toys, objects, or schedules.
- spends a lot of time lining things up or putting things in a certain order.

Three groups are at higher risk for ASD, including: boys (male: female ration 4:1), siblings of those with autism (risk for subsequent occurrence is 5%–6%), and people with certain other developmental disorders such as FXS, DS, or tuberous sclerosis. The majority of cases have no clear etiology. Reported prevalence of ASD in North America is 6 per 1,000.[31]

Prognosis depends on many factors and is difficult to predict. Important factors include level of cognitive functioning, the presence of epilepsy or other medical co-morbidities, attention and functional play skills. Favorable factors include early identification and appropriate behavioral intervention, and successful inclusion with typically-developing peers in mainstream educational and community settings. Poorer outcomes are associated with the presence of ID, epilepsy, no functional use of language by five years, co-morbid medical/genetic conditions and psychiatric disorders.[20,42]

Although there is no cure or one single treatment for autism spectrum disorders, there are ways to minimize the symptoms and maximize learning.

- Behavioral and other therapeutic options.[12,24]
- Educational and school-based options
- Medication options - The U.S. FDA has not approved any medications specifically for the treatment of autism, but in many cases medication can treat some of the associated symptoms. Selective serotonin reuptake inhibitors, tricyclics, psychoactive/anti-psychotics, stimulants, and anti-anxiety drugs are among the medications used.
- Individualized, success-oriented programs will improve strength, balance, motor planning, etc., and decrease frequency of self-stimulating behaviors and response to sensory information.

Fetal Alcohol Syndrome

Fetal Alcohol Spectrum Disorders (FASD) describes the range of effects that can occur in an individual whose mother drank alcohol during pregnancy. The fetal brain is particularly sensitive to alcohol, which passes through the placenta into the developing baby, during the period of rapid growth in the third trimester. The effects may include physical, mental, behavioral, and/or learning disabilities with possible lifelong implications. People affected by FASD can have brain damage; facial deformities; growth deficits; mental retardation; heart, lung and kidney defects; hyperactivity; attention and memory problems; poor coordination; behavioral problems; and learning disabilities.[10,21,37,46]

The diagnosis of fetal alcohol syndrome (FAS) is based on four criteria:

(1) prenatal alcohol exposure (confirmed or unconfirmed)
(2) growth retardation (height and weight < 10th percentile)
(3) facial characteristics (smoothing of groove above upper lip, small palpebral fissures (separation of upper and lower eyelids)
(4) neurodevelopment problems (poor coordination, visual motor difficulties, nystagmus, or difficulty with motor control)

One of the following central nervous system abnormalities is also usually present:

(1) Structural abnormalities including head circumference at or below the 10th percentile, and observation of abnormal brain structure from image studies.

(2) Functional abnormalities evidenced by either global cognitive or intellectual deficits, or functional deficits. Global cognitive or intellectual deficits are below the third percentile or two standard deviations below the mean for standardized testing. Functional deficits are below the sixteenth percentile in at least three of the following: cognitive or developmental deficits, executive functioning, motor functioning delay, problems with attention or hyperactivity, poor social skills, or others (such as sensory problems, memory deficits)

There are many long-term effects of FAS. The majority of adults have problems leading independent lives. Many young adults who do not receive appropriate support are unable to maintain continuous education, employment and relationships. Additionally, many have legal problems. Common areas of concern include: distractibility, easily frustrated, poor fine and gross motor skills, poor attention, lack of organizational skills, problems with concrete thinking, and poor peer relations.[15, 34]

General Risks in all Groups with ID

The Special Olympics (SO) Healthy Athletes program has documented that low bone density (osteopenia/osteoporosis) occurs in about one-fifth of all Special Olympics athletes (average age, 24 years). While the causes are not completely known, this might be attributed to medications, lack of physical activity, or metabolic condition.[48] Low bone density is correlated with an increased risk of bone fracture. A t-score (rating of bone density) of -1 or lower is considered osteopenic. A t-score of -1.5 is roughly four times more likely to be associated with a bone fracture than a t-score of 0.[6] Hence, it is plausible that fracture risk would be higher in this population, and especially in those taking at-risk medications. In a recent unpublished program evaluation of SO athletes, 31% of athletes were taking medications which could induce low bone density. Athletes taking these medications had an average t-score of -0.6., while athletes not taking medications which induce low bone density as a side effect had an average t-score of 0.0.[47]

Some types of ID are associated with collagen and bone abnormalities, as well as structural abnormalities of the spine, joints and limbs which can also place the person at risk.

Seizure disorders occur in roughly 26% of people with ID.[14] Many anti-seizure medications have behavioral side effects which may conflict with best performance.[48] Those interested in any sports involving water, heights or high speeds should have a seizure disorder under control before they engage. Additionally, compliance with medication regimens should be stressed.

Many types of ID are associated with metabolic abnormalities, thyroid or kidney disorders, thermoregulation disorders, or differences in pain perception, any of which may predispose to heat stroke or electrolyte disturbances. Any special circumstances that may increase metabolic risk should be noted, and attention to diet, proper hydration and exercise self-monitoring should be fostered.

Medical Management

Federal legislation entitles children with ID to free testing and appropriate, individualized education and skills training within the school system from ages 3 to 21. For children under the age of 3, many states have early intervention programs. Many schools help train children in basic skills such as bathing and feeding. Most children attend school, although children with more significant needs may require a specialized program. Some high school graduates can participate in post-secondary education, and many adults are capable of working in the community, some in a more structured environment.

Training in independent living and job skills is often begun in early adulthood. Mildly involved individuals can often acquire the skills needed to live independently and hold a job. Moderate to profoundly involved individuals usually require supervised community living. A supportive environment is essential to help those with ID reach their full potential.

Medications

Because of the variety of causes and medical problems specific to those with ID, Special Olympics has developed a Medication Watch List for individuals with ID. This list is available online and guides the practitioner regarding the medication along with possible side effects. Download the list at http://media.specialolympics.org/soi/files/healthy-athletes/MedFest_Medical_Watch_list.doc.

Special Considerations

The following suggestions can assist the development of successful programming for any person with ID:

- Be aware of the need to modify the task or protocol for the individual situation
- Simplify the task and instructions — have them perform one task at a time.
- If the activity is new, walk through it first to familiarize them with the activity
- To make sure they understand, have them repeat the instructions.
- Allow short breaks when necessary.
- Provide simple descriptions with pictures and few words in larger font
- Assess amount of effort using visual scales, like the ACSM modified BORG scale
- Consider group activities and family involvement
- Be prepared for inconsistent performance, frustration and individual attention.
- Encourage practice and repetition to offset poor memory.
- They may not be able to generalize information they have learned from one day to the next. It is important to make eye contact, repeat things and use short instructions.

- Encourage success and reward positive behavior with praise or incentives. Positive reinforcement should be immediate.
- Concepts that may be problematic include decision-making, time, impulsiveness and distinguishing between public and private behaviors
- Create borders to help them feel more secure and calm.
- If behavior problems occur, defuse the situation calmly and move into a new activity.
- Using visual, concrete examples and hands-on learning is easier
- As some may have trouble expressing themselves, be aware of body language and know warning signs for frustration, sadness, anger and other hurtful emotions.

Chapter 20, Part I References

1. American Association on Intellectual and Developmental Disabilities (2010). Assessed at http://www.aaidd.org/content_100.cfm&navID=21

2. Ali, F.E., Al-Bustan, M.A., Al-Busairi, W.A., Al-Mulla, F.A., Esbaita, E.Y. (2006). Cervical spine abnormalities associated with Down syndrome. International Orthopaedics, 30(4):284-9. Epub 2006 Mar 7.

3. Arron, K., Oliver, C., Moss, J., Berg, K., Burbidge, C. (2010). The prevalence and phenomenology of self-injurious and aggressive behaviour in genetic syndromes. Journal Intellectual Disability Research.. doi: 10.1111/j.1365-2788.2010.01337.x. [Epub ahead of print]

4. Braganza SF. (2003). Atlantoaxial dislocation. Pediatric Reviews, 24(3):106-7; discussion 106-7.

5. Armatas, V. (2009). Mental retardation: definitions, etiology, epidemiology anddiagnosis. Journal of Sport and Health Research., 1(2):112-122.

6. Consensus Development Conference, 1993. American Journal of Medicine 1993; 94:646-650. Available at http://www.medscape.com/viewarticle/410799_2

7. Croen, L.A., Grether, J.K., & Selvin, S. (2001). The Epidemiology of Mental Retardation of Unknown Cause. Pediatrics, 107(6):E86

8. Daily, D.K., Ardinger, H.H., & Holmes, G.E. (2000a).Identificationand evaluation of mental retardation. American Family Physician, 62(5):961-963.

9. Daily, D.K., Ardinger, H.H., & Holmes, G.E. (2000b). Identificationand evaluation of mental retardation. American Family Physician, 61(4):1059-1067.

10. Dalen, K., Bruarøy, S., Wentzel-Larsen, T., Laegreid, L.M. (2009). Cognitive functioning in children prenatally exposed to alcholo and psychotrophic drugs. Neuropediatrics, 40(4):162-7. Epub 2010 Feb 4

11. Dennis J, Archer N, Ellis J, Marder L. (2010)/ Recognizing heart disease in children with Down syndrome. Archives Disease Child Education and Practices Ed, 95(4):98-104.

12. Devlin, S., Healy, O., Leader, G., Hughes, B.M. (2010). Comparison of Behavioral Intervention and Sensory-Integration Therapy in the Treatment of Challenging Behavior. Journal Autism Developmental Disorders. 2010, Dec 10. (Epub ahead of print).

13. Englund, H., Annerén, G., Gustafsson, J., Wester, U., Wiltfang, J., Lannfelt, L., Blennow, K., Höglund, K. (2007). Increase in beta-amyloid levels in cerebrospinal fluid of children with Down syndrome. Dementia Geriatric Cognitive Disorders, 24(5):369-74. Epub 2007 Oct 3

14. Epilepsy Foundation Online. Available at: http://www.efwp.org/programs/side_effects.shtml. Accessed June 23, 2007.

15. Freunscht, I., Feldmann, R. (2010). Young Adults with Fetal Alcohol Syndrome (FAS): Social, Emotional and Occupational Development. Klinische Pädiatrie. 2010, July 30. (Epub ahead of print).

16. Fudge, J.C. Jr, Li, S., Jaggers, J., O'Brien, S.M., Peterson, E.D., Jacobs, J.P., Welke, K.F., Jacobs, M.L., Li, J.S., Pasquali, S.K. (2010). Congenital heart surgery outcomes in Down syndrome: analysis of a national clinical database. Pediatrics, 126(2):315-22. Epub 2010 Jul 12.

17. Hagerman R, Hoem G, Hagerman P. (2010). Fragile X and autism: Intertwined at the molecular level leading to targeted treatments. Molecular Autism, 21;1(1):12

18. Haqq, A,M., Muehlbauer, M.J., Newgard, C.B., Grambow, S., Freemark, M. (2010). The Metabolic Phenotype of Prader-Willi Syndrome (PWS) in Childhood: Heightened Insulin Sensitivity Relative to Body Mass Index. *Journal Clinical Endocrinology Metabolism.* 2010, Oct 20. [Epub ahead of print]

19. Hankinson, T.C., & Anderson, R.C. (2010). Craniovertebral junction abnormalities in Down syndrome. *Neurosurgery,* 66(3 Suppl):32-8.

20. Johnson CP, Myers SM; American Academy of Pediatrics Council on Children With Disabilities.(2007). Identification and evaluation of children with autism spectrum disorders. *Pediatrics,* Nov;120(5):1183-215. Epub 2007 Oct 29. Review.

21. Jones KL, Hoyme HE, Robinson LK, Del Campo M, Manning MA, Prewitt LM, Chambers CD. (2010). Fetal alcohol spectrum disorders: Extending the range of structural defects. *American Journal Medical Genetics A,* 152A(11):2731-5.

22. Kolevzon, A., Gross, R., & Reichenberg, A. (2007). Prenatal and Perinatal Risk Factors for Autism: A Review and Integration of Findings. Archives Pediatric Adolescent Medicine, 161(4):326-333.

23. Krinsky-McHale,S.J., Devenny, D.A., Kittler, P., Silverman, W. (2008). Selective attention deficits associated with mild cognitive impairment and early stage Alzheimer's disease in adults with Down syndrome. *American Journal Mental Retardation,* 113(5):369-86

24. Landa, R.J, Holman, K.C, O'Neill, A.H, Stuart, E.A. (2011). Intervention targeting development of socially synchronous engagement in toddlers with autism spectrum disorder: a randomized controlled trial. *Journal Child Psychology Psychiatry.* 2011 Jan;52(1):13-21. doi: 10.1111/j.1469-7610.2010.02288.x. Epub 2010 Dec 3

25. Leonard, H., & Xingyan Wen, X. (2002). The epidemiology of mental retardation: Challenges andopportunities in the newmillennium. *Mental Retardation and Developmental Disabilities Research Reviews,* 8(3):117-134.

26. Martínez-Quintana E, Rodríguez-González F, Medina-Gil JM, Agredo-Muñoz J, Nieto-Lago V. (2010). Clinical outcome in Down syndrome patients with congenital heart disease. *Cir Cir,* 78(3):245-50.

27. McAllister, C.J., Whittington, J.E., Holland, A.J. (2010). Development of the eating behaviour in Prader-Willi Syndrome: advances in our understanding. *International Journal Obesity.* 2010, Aug 3. (Epub ahead of print).

28. McDuffie A., Abbeduto, L., Lewis, P., Kover, S., Kim, J.S., Weber, A., Brown, W.T. (2010). Autism spectrum disorder in children and adolescents with fragile X syndrome: within-syndrome differences and age-related changes. *American Journal Intellectual Developmental Disabilities,* 115(4):307-26.

29. Miles, J. H., McCathren, R.B., Stichter, J., Shinawi, M. Autism Spectrum Disorders. In: Pagon RA, Bird TC, Dolan CR, Stephens K, editors. GeneReviews [Internet]. Seattle (WA): University of Washington, Seattle; 1993-.2003 Aug 27 [updated 2010 Apr 13].

30. National Association for Down syndrome http://www.nads.org/

31. National Autism Association http://www.nationalautismassociation.org/#

32. National Institutes of Health, E. K. Shriver National Institute of Child Health and Human Development, 2010. http://www.nichd.nih.gov/health/topics/asd.cfm

33. National Fragile X Foundation http://www.nfxf.org/html/home.shtml

34. National Organization of Fetal Alcohol Syndrome http://www.nofas.org/healthcare/

35. National Prader Willi Association

36. Nieuwenhuis-Mark RE. (2009). Diagnosing Alzheimer's dementia in Down syndrome: problems and possible solutions. *Research Developmental Disabilities.* Sep-Oct;30(5):827-38. Epub 2009 Mar 6. Review

37. O'Leary CM, Nassar N, Kurinczuk JJ, de Klerk N, Geelhoed E, Elliott EJ, Bower C. Prenatal alcohol exposure and risk of birth defects. *Pediatrics.* 2010 Oct; 126(4):e843-50. Epub 2010 Sep 27

38. Prader Willi Association. http://www.pwsausa.org/

39. Platt, L.S. (2001). Medical and orthopaedic conditions in Special Olympics athletes. *Journal Athletic Training,* 36(1):74-80.

40. Raspa M, Bailey DB, Bishop E, Holiday D, Olmsted M. (2010). Obesity, food selectivity, and physical activity in individuals with fragile X syndrome. *American Journal Intellectual Developmental Disability* 115(6), 482-495.

41. Schalock, R.L., Luckasson, R.A., and Shogren K.A. (2007). "Perspectives: The Renaming of Mental Retardation: Understanding the Change to the Term Intellectual Disability," *Intellectual and Developmental Disabilities.* 45:2 (2007): 116-124

42. Turner LM, Stone WL, Pozdol SL, Coonrod EE. (2006). Follow-up of children with autism spectrum disorders from age 2 to age 9. *Autism,* May;10(3):243-65.

43. REUS L, ZWARTS M, VAN VLIMMEREN LA, WILLEMSEN MA, OTTEN BJ, NIJHUIS-VAN DER SANDEN MW. (2011). (2011). MOTOR PROBLEMS IN PRADER-WILLI SYNDROME: A SYSTEMATIC REVIEW ON BODY COMPOSITION AND NEUROMUSCULAR FUNCTIONING. *NEUROSCIENCE BIOBEHAVORIAL REVIEW*, 35(3):956-69. EPUB 2010 NOV 4.

44. RAO S, SALMON G. (2010). AUTISM SPECTRUM DISORDERS. *BRITISH JOURNAL HOSPITAL MEDICINE* (LONDON), 71(12):699-703

45. STRØMME, P., & HAGBERG, G. (2007). AETIOLOGY IN SEVERE AND MILD MENTAL RETARDATION: A POPULATION-BASED STUDY OF NORWEGIAN CHILDREN. *DEVELOPMENTAL MEDICINE & CHILD NEUROLOGY*, 42(2):76-86.

46. REHM J, BALIUNAS D, BORGES GL, GRAHAM K, IRVING H, KEHOE T, PARRY CD, PATRA J, POPOVA S, POZNYAK V, ROERECKE M, ROOM R, SAMOKHVALOV AV, TAYLOR B. (2010). THE RELATION BETWEEN DIFFERENT DIMENSIONS OF ALCHOLO CONSUMPTION AND BURDEN OF DISEASE: AN OVERVIEW. *ADDICTION*, 105(5):817-43. EPUB 2010 MAR 15

47. SPECIAL OLYMPICS, INC. ONLINE. AVAILABLE AT: HTTP://WWW.SPECIALOLYMPICS.ORG/NR/RDONLYRES/44/EOIH4KZWS56HFY3T4X7AGK7W6YQTUKYU65WLS2N4NKQG3XRZ5TZQY32G3SMTTCZ7MA2ZB22MSFH4OE56TUALSLREDQC/BONE_DENSITY.PDF. ACCESSED JUNE 18, 2007.

48. SPECIAL OLYMPICS MEDFEST, 2007. ASSESSED AT HTTP://MEDIA.SPECIALOLYMPICS.ORG/SOI/FILES/HEALTHYATHLETES/MEDFEST%20MANUAL%202010.PDF

49. UNITED STATES DEPARTMENT OF EDUCATION. (2006). TWENTY-SIXTH ANNUAL REPORT TO CONGRESS ON THE IMPLEMENTATION OF THE INDIVIDUALS WITH DISABILITIES EDUCATION ACT, PARTS B AND C. ASSESSED AT HTTP://WWW2.ED.GOV/ABOUT/REPORTS/ANNUAL/OSEP/2006/PARTS-B-C/INDEX.HTML

50. ZIGMAN WB, LOTT IT. (2007). ALZHEIMER'S DISEASE IN DOWN SYNDROME: NEUROBIOLOGY RISK. *MENTAL RETARDATION DEVELOPMENTAL DISABILITIES RESEARCH REVIEW*, 13(3):237-46.

51. ZOGHBI HY. (2003). POSTNATAL NEURODEVELOPMENTAL DISORDERS: MEETING AT THE SYNAPSE? *SCIENCE*, OCT 31;302(5646):826-30

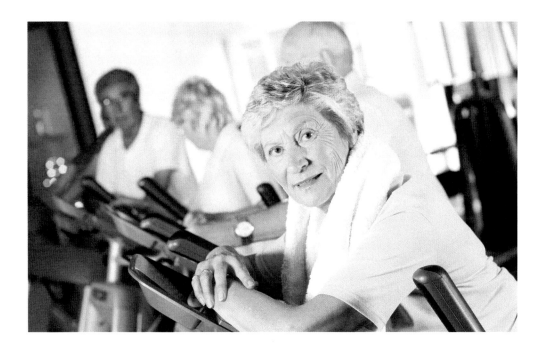

PART II
DEMENTIAS

Overview of the Condition

Dementia is a general term that describes a group of symptoms caused by disorders that affect the brain. People with dementia have memory loss and impaired intellectual functioning that interferes with normal activities and relationships. They can lose their ability to problem solve and maintain emotional control. They may experience changes in personality and behavioral problems such as agitation and delusions. A diagnosis of dementia is made when two or more functions of the brain (*i.e.*, memory, language skills, or cognitive skills) are significantly impaired.

Dementia can be primary, not resulting from another disease (*i.e.*, Alzheimer disease); or secondary, resulting from a physical disease or injury such as stroke.[35] Alzheimer disease is the most common type of dementia, accounting for 60% to 80% of all cases of dementia in those over the age of 65. Vascular dementia is the second most common type. Other causes for dementia include:

- Lewy body dementia
- Frontotemporal dementia
- HIV-associated dementia
- Huntington's disease
- Dementia pugilistica
- Corticobasal degeneration
- Creutzfeldt-Jakob disease

• Other rare hereditary dementias

Mild cognitive impairment (MCI) is a condition in which a person has problems with memory, language, or other mental functions that are noticeable to others and on tests, but not serious enough to interfere with daily life. Although those with MCI are at greater risk for progression to Alzheimer disease, not all people with MCI do advance.[7,17,20,28]

Alzheimer disease

Named after Dr. Alois Alzheimer, who first recognized the disease in 1906, Alzheimer disease (AD) is an irreversible, progressive brain disease that slowly destroys memory and thinking skills, and eventually the ability to carry out tasks. Experts suggest that as many as 5.1 million Americans may have AD.

In most people, symptoms first appear after the age of 60 years. The prevalence increases exponentially > 65 years; about 13% of people older than 65 and approximately 50% of those > 80 years will be diagnosed with this type of dementia. Studies have linked a gene called APOE to this late-onset AD. One form of the gene, APOE 4, increases a person's risk of getting the disease; about 40% of people who develop late-onset AD carry this gene. However, carrying this gene does not necessarily mean that a person will develop AD, and people carrying no APOE 4 forms can also develop the disease.[5] A few people develop AD in their 30s, 40s, or 50s; many of these people have a mutation in a gene that they inherited from a parent. These gene mutations cause AD in these "early-onset" familial cases, but not all early-onset cases are caused by such mutations.[8,14,21]

Gender differences have been observed — 16% of women older than 71 years have dementia, while only 11% of men of the same age group do. The difference may have more to do with the greater longevity of women than with gender-based propensity.[3] In

FIGURE 20.1

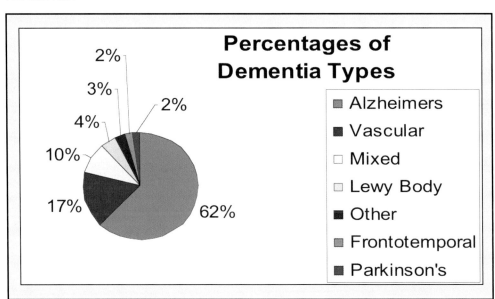

Table 20.2 Drug Management [2]

Name (actual/generic) or class	Purpose	Common Side Effects	Exercise/Activity Cautions
Cholinesterase Inhibitors (Aricept, Exelon, and Razadyne or Reminal)	Prevent breakdown of acetylcholine to maintain nerve cell communication	Nausea, vomiting, loss of appetite, increased frequency of bowel movements	• Monitor personal comfort. • Check for pain, hunger, thirst, constipation, full bladder, fatigue, infections and skin irritation. • Maintain comfortable room temperature. • Avoid being confrontational or arguing; respond to the feeling behind what's being expressed. • Redirect the person's attention. • Remain flexible, patient and supportive.
Mamentine (Namenda)	Regulates activity of glutamate, a chemical involved in learning and memory.	Headache, constipation, confusion and dizziness.	• Create a calm environment. Avoid noise, glare, insecure space, and background distraction, including television. • Simplify the environment, tasks and solutions. • Allow adequate rest between events. • Maintain constant attendance so person does not wander or feel lost.
Antidepressants (Celexa, Prozac, Paxil, Zoloft, Desyrel)	Low mood and irritability		• Stop the exercise if client becomes overly fatigued or short of breath; discuss the symptoms with MD or schedule an appointment for evaluation. • Do not exercise if client is not feeling well or has a fever. Wait a few days after all symptoms disappear before restarting the exercise program, unless MD gives other directions. • If client experiences shortness of breath or increased fatigue during any activity, slow down or stop the activity. Elevate the feet when resting. If client continues to have shortness of breath, call MD. The MD may make changes in medications, diet, or fluid restrictions. • Stop the activity if client develops a rapid or irregular heartbeat or has heart palpitations. Check pulse after rest for 15 minutes. If it's still above 120-150 beats per minute, call the MD for further instructions
Anxiolytics (Ativan, Serax)	Anxiety, restlessness, verbally disruptive behavior and resistance:	Drowsiness, sleepiness, fatigue, poor coordination, unsteadiness, behavior changes	
Antipsychotics (Abilify, Clozaril, Haldol, Zyprexa, Seroquel, Risperdal, Geodon)	Hallucinations, delusions, agitation, aggression, hostility, uncooperative behavior	Weight gain, drowsiness, difficulty swallowing, hyperlipidemia, diabetes, prolonged QTC interval, myocarditis, extrapyramidal symptoms, cataract, lower life expectancy with long-term use	• Exercise caution in situations that raise body temperature (strenuous exercise, hot weather), as meds may interfere with the body's ability to control core temperature; • Check heart rate frequently for arrhythmias • Be aware of symptoms of stroke, as several meds increase the risk of cerebrovascular events, such as stroke, in elderly patients with dementia-related psychosis
Seizure Medications (Tegretol, Depakote)	Stabilize mood	**Tegretol:** Dizziness, drowsiness, blurred or double vision, nausea, skin rashes. **Depakote:** Upset stomach, altered bleeding time, liver toxicity, hair loss, weight gain, tremor	• Avoid becoming overheated or dehydrated during exercise and in hot weather. • Follow your doctor's instructions about the type and amount of liquids you should drink. In some cases, drinking too much liquid can be as unsafe as not drinking enough

addition, differences between racial/ethnic groups within the United States have been documented. The rates of dementia may be higher among African-Americans than among whites.

Research also links the disease to lifestyle-related factors, such as obesity, diabetes, high blood pressure, and high cholesterol.[9,12,13,24,29] As African-Americans have higher rates of high blood pressure and type 2 diabetes, this may account for the higher prevalence of AD. People with a history of depression also appear more vulnerable. AD is less common among the highly educated, a possible beneficial consequence of learning and use of memory among those with more education.[25,27,42]

AD is characterized by several abnormalities in the brain: amyloid plaques and neurofibrillary tangles. The brain begins to churn out amyloid that is initially a long protein. However, the amyloid is cut by enzymes into shorter pieces that become sticky and clump together, forming plaques. Once plaques form, the tau protein that maintains structural integrity of the neural network breaks down, interrupting electrical signals along the nerve. Nerve cells begin to die, leaving tangled debris. This debris stimulates the immune system which responds with inflammation to remove the debris. Researchers are not sure if plaques and tangles are in themselves harmful or merely side effects of a disease process that damages neurons and leads to symptoms. However, the plaques and tangles usually increase as AD progresses.[2,6,43]

In the early stages, patients may experience impairment of memory, lapses of judgment, and subtle changes in personality. As the disorder progresses, memory and language problems worsen; patients begin to have difficulty performing activities of daily living, such as balancing a checkbook or remembering medications. They also may have visual-spatial problems, such as difficulty with an unfamiliar driving route. They may become disoriented about place and time, may suffer delusions (*i.e.,* the idea that someone is stealing things), and may become short-tempered or hostile. During late stages, patients lose the ability to control motor functions; they may have difficulty swallowing and lose bowel and bladder control. They eventually do not recognize family members and lose the ability to speak. The disease then begins to affect the emotions and behavior, and eventually symptoms such as aggression, agitation, depression, sleeplessness develop.[23]

On average, patients with AD live for eight to 10 years after diagnosis; however, some people live as long as 20 years. Patients with AD often die of aspiration pneumonia because they lose the ability to swallow.[45]

Currently, there is no cure for AD. Treatments, both drug (See Table 20.2) and non-drug, manage symptoms and may slow the progression.[15,33]

Non-Drug Management

Successful non-drug treatments include:
- Recognizing that the person is having symptoms, not just being mean or ornery.
- Understanding how a symptom may relate to the experience of the person.
- Changing the person's environment to resolve challenges and obstacles, and increase security and peace of mind.

Anyone who develops behavioral symptoms should have a thorough medical exam, especially if symptoms appear suddenly. Even if the cause is AD, other treatable conditions that contribute to the behavior may be revealed in the exam.

Vascular Dementia

This is the second most common cause of dementia, accounting for 20% of all dementias, and may coexist with Alzheimer disease. It is caused by brain damage from cerebrovascular or cardiovascular problems — usually stroke.[10,18,26] It may also result from genetic diseases or endocarditis (infection of a heart valve). The incidence of vascular dementia increases with advancing age and is similar in men and women.

Symptoms of vascular dementia may begin suddenly. Patients may have a history of high blood pressure, vascular disease, previous strokes or heart attack. Vascular dementia may or may not get worse with time; in some cases, symptoms may get better. When the disease does get worse, it has a stepwise progression with sudden changes in ability. Unlike people with Alzheimer disease, people with vascular dementia often maintain their personality and normal emotional responsiveness until later stages. People with vascular dementia often wander at night and have other problems commonly found in people who have had a stroke, including depression and incontinence.

There are several types of vascular dementia, varying in cause and symptoms. One type, multi-infarct dementia (MID), is caused by numerous small strokes that cause multiple damaged areas, along with extensive lesions in the white matter, or nerve fibers, of the brain. Because the damage in MID affect isolated areas of the brain, the symptoms are often limited to one side of the body, or may affect one or a few specific functions, such as language. Although not all strokes cause dementia, a single stroke can damage the brain enough to cause dementia; this condition is called single-infarct dementia. Dementia is more common when the stroke takes place on the left side of the brain and/or when it involves the hippocampus, a structure important for memory. If the damage is in the mid-brain region, the dementia has a gradual, progressive impairment that looks like Alzheimer disease.[39,41]

Other causes of vascular dementia include vasculitis, inflammation of the blood vessel system; profound low blood pressure; or lesions caused by bleeding in the brain. Lupus erythematosis, an autoimmune disease and temporal arteritis, an inflammatory disease, can also damage blood vessels and lead to vascular dementia.

There is no standard drug treatment for vascular dementia, although medications can be used to treat some of the symptoms (*i.e.,* depression). Most treatments try to reduce risk factors for further brain damage. Medications to relieve restlessness or depression or to aid sleep better may also be prescribed. Some studies have noted that cholinesterase inhibitors can improve cognitive function and behavioral symptoms in patients with early vascular dementia.

The progression of vascular dementia can often be slowed or stopped if the underlying vascular risk factors are treated. To prevent strokes and transient ischemic attacks, medicines to control high blood pressure, high cholesterol, heart disease, and diabetes may be prescribed. Sometimes aspirin, warfarin, or other drugs that prevent clots from forming in small blood vessels are prescribed.[31] If patients have blockage of a blood vessel, surgical procedures, such as carotid endarterectomy, stenting, or angioplasty, may restore normal blood supply.

Special Precautions

If the client is on medications to prevent blood clotting, they may bleed more easily. Caution must be taken to avoid injury while exercising.

Continuous monitoring of blood pressure before, during and after exercise is also indicated to avoid episodes of high or increased BP. Care should also be taken to avoid any Valsalva maneuvers while exercising through constant steady breathing.

If the client has diabetes, continual monitoring of blood glucose for hypo or hyperglycemia is necessary. A container of juice, honey, or glucose tablets should be kept on hand for hypoglycemia episodes.

Ways to prevent or delay the onset of dementia

(1) **Healthy eating**[16,30]
   - Lower homocysteine: Elevated levels of the amino acid homocysteine were associated with a 2.9 times greater risk of Alzheimer disease and a 4.9 times greater risk of vascular dementia.[38] Studies have shown that high doses of three B vitamins that help lower homocysteine levels — folic acid, B12, and B6 — appear to slow the progression of Alzheimer disease.[34]
   - Lower cholesterol levels: Research has suggested that people with high cholesterol levels have an increased risk of developing Alzheimer disease. Cholesterol is involved in formation of amyloid plaques in the brain. Mutations in a gene called CYP46 and the APOE E4 gene variant, both of which have been linked to an increased risk of Alzheimer disease, are also involved in cholesterol metabolism. Several studies have also found that the use of drugs called statins, which lower cholesterol levels, is associated with a lower likelihood of cognitive impairment.[40]

(2) **Lower blood pressure:** Several studies have shown that antihypertensive medicine reduces the odds of cognitive impairment in elderly people with high blood pressure.[32,36,37] These people had a reduced risk of both Alzheimer disease and vascular dementia.

(3) **Exercise:** Regular exercise stimulates production of chemicals called growth factors that help neurons survive and adapt to new situations. These gains may help to delay the onset of dementia symptoms. Exercise also may reduce the risk of brain damage from atherosclero-

sis.[1,4,19,22]

(4) Education and Cognitive Activity: Researchers have found evidence that formal education may help protect people against the effects of Alzheimer disease. In one study, researchers found that people with more years of formal education had relatively less mental decline than people with less schooling, regardless of the number of amyloid plaques and neurofibrillary tangles each person had in his or her brain. Researchers think education and continued cognitive activity may cause the brain to develop robust nerve cell networks that help compensate for the cell damage caused by Alzheimer disease.[11,44]

Special Considerations

The following suggestions can assist the development of successful programming for a person with dementia:

- Individualize the activity and program for each person daily.
- Perform the program in an environment that is safe and familiar.
- Simplify and demonstrate the task.
- Perform one task at a time.
- Video, television, and music have been demonstrated to assist programming.
- Use structured routines that become familiar to reduce stress.
- Utilize short exercise periods interspersed with short breaks.
- Consider group activities and family involvement.
- Be prepared for inconsistent performance and attention.
- Information may not be retained from day to day, so repetition may be necessary.
- Reward positive behavior immediately with praise or incentives.
- If behavior problems occur, move into a new activity.
- Since emotional expression may be compromised, be aware of body language and warning signs for frustration, sadness, anger and other emotions.

Chapter 20, Part II References

1. Aarsland D., Sardahaee F.S., Anderssen S., Ballard C., and Alzheimer's Society Systematic Review group. (2010). Is physical activity a potential preventive factor for vascular dementia? A systematic review. *Aging Mental Health*, 14(4), 386-95.

2. Alzheimer's Association (2010). http://www.alz.org/index.asp

3. Azad N.A., Al Bugami M., Loy-English I. (2007). Gender differences in dementia risk factors. *Gender Medicine*, 4(2),120-9.

4. Baker L.D., Frank L.L., Foster-Schubert K., Green P.S., Wilkinson C.W., McTiernan A., Plymate S.R., Fishel M.A., Watson G.S., Cholerton B.A., Duncan G.E., Mehta P.D., Craft S. (2010). Effects of aerobic exercise on mild cognitive impairment: a controlled trial. *Archives Neurology*, 67(1), 71-9.

5. Bookheimer S., Burggren A. (2009). APOE-4 genotype and neurophysiological vulnerability to Alzheimer's and cognitive aging. *Annual Review Clinical Psychology*, 5,343-62.

6. Braak, H., Rüb, U., Schultz, C., Del Tredici, K. (2006). Vulnerability of cortical neurons to Alzheimer's and Parkinson's diseases. Journal Alzheimers Disease, 9(3 Suppl), 35-44.

7. Busse, A., Hensel, A., Gühne, U., Angermeyer, M.C., Riedel-Heller, S.G. (2006). Mild cognitive impairment: long-term course of four clinical subtypes. Neurology, 67(12):2176-85.

8. Chai C.K. (2007). The genetics of Alzheimer's disease. American Journal Alzheimers Disease Other Dementias, 22(1):37-41.

9. Chen J.H., Lin K.P., Chen Y.C. (2009). Risk factors for dementia. Journal Formosa Medical Association, 108(10):754-64.

10. Cherubini A., Lowenthal D.T., Paran E., Mecocci P., Williams L.S., Senin U. (2010). Hypertension and cognitive function in the elderly. Disease Monthly, 56(3):106-47.

11. Daffner K.R. (2010). Promoting successful cognitive aging: a comprehensive review. Journal Alzheimers Disease, 19(4):1101-22

12. Dickstein D.L., Walsh J., Brautigam H., Stockton S.D. Jr, Gandy S., Hof, P.R. (2010).

13. Role of vascular risk factors and vascular dysfunction in Alzheimer's disease. Mt Sinai Journal Medicine, 77(1),82-102.

14. Ertekin-Taner N. (2007). Genetics of Alzheimer's disease: a centennial review. Neurology Clinics, 25(3):611-67, v.

15. Fillit, H.M., Doody, R.S., Binaso, K., Crook,,G.M., Ferris, S.H., Farlow, M.R., Leifer, B., Mills, C., Minkoff, N., Orland, B., Reichman, W.E., Salloway, S. (2006). Recommendations for best practices in the treatment of Alzheimer's disease in managed care. American Journal Geriatric Pharmacotherapy, 4 Suppl A:S9-S24; quiz S25-S28.

16. Féart C., Samieri C., Barberger-Gateau P. (2010). Mediterranean diet and cognitive function in older adults. Current Opinions Clinical Nutrition Metabolic Care, 13(1),14-8.

17. Gauthier, S., Reisberg, B., Zaudig, M., Petersen, R.C., Ritchie, K., Broich, K., Belleville, S., Brodaty, H., Bennett ,D,, Chertkow, H., Cummings, J.L., de Leon, M., Feldman, H., Ganguli, M., Hampel H., Scheltens, P., Tierney, M.C., Whitehouse, P., Winblad, B.; International Psychogeriatric Association Expert Conference on mild cognitive impairment. (2006). Mild cognitive impairment. Lancet, 367(9518),1262-70.

18. Gold ,G., Kovari, E., Hof ,P.R., Bouras, C., Giannakopoulos ,P. (2007). Sorting out the clinical consequences of ischemic lesions in brain aging: a clinicopathological approach. Journal Neurological Science, 257(1-2),17-22. Epub 2007 Feb 23.

19. Lee Y., Back J.H., Kim J., Kim S.H., Na D.L., Cheong H.K., Hong C.H., Kim Y.G. (2010). Systematic review of health behavioral risks and cognitive health in older adults. International Psychogeriatrics, 22(2), 174-87. Epub 2009 Nov 3.

20. Levey, A., Lah, J., Goldstein, F., Steenland, K., Bliwise, D. (2006). Mild cognitive impairment: an opportunity to identify patients at high risk for progression to Alzheimer's disease. Clinical Therapies, 28(7):991-1001.

21. Mendez MF. (2006). The accurate diagnosis of early-onset dementia. International Journal Psychiatry Medicine, 36(4),401-12.

22. Middleton LE, Yaffe K. (2009). Promising strategies for the prevention of dementia. Archives Neurology, 66(10),1210-5.

23. Mitchell S.L., Teno J.M., Kiely D.K., Shaffer M.L., Jones R.N., Prigerson H.G., Volicer L., Givens J.L., Hamel M.B. (2009). The clinical course of advanced dementia. New England Journal Medicine, 361(16),1529-38.

24. Naderali E.K., Ratcliffe S.H., Dale M.C. (2009). Obesity and Alzheimer's disease: a link between body weight and cognitive function in old age. American Journal Alzheimers Disease Other Dementias, 24(6):445-9.

25. Paradise M., Cooper C., Livingston G. (2009). Systematic review of the effect of education on survival in Alzheimer's disease. International Psychogeriatrics, 21(1),25-32. Epub 2008 Nov 25.

26. Pendlebury S.T., Rothwell P.M. (2009). Prevalence, incidence, and factors associated with pre-stroke and post-stroke dementia: a systematic review and meta-analysis. Lancet Neurology, 8(11):1006-18. Epub 2009 Sep 24.

27. Peters R., Beckett N., Forette F., Tuomilehto J., Ritchie C., Walton I., Waldman A., Clarke R., Poulter R., Fletcher A., Bulpitt C. (2009). Vascular risk factors and cognitive function among 3763 participants in the Hypertension in the Very Elderly Trial (HYVET): a cross-sectional analysis. International Psychogeriatrics, 21(2):359-68. Epub 2009 Feb 27.

28. Petersen, R.C., Negash, S. (2008). Mild cognitive impairment: an overview. CNS Spectrum, 13(1),45-53.

29. Profenno L.A., Porsteinsson A.P., Faraone S.V. (2010). Meta-analysis of Alzheimer's disease risk with obesity, diabetes, and related disorders. Biological Psychiatry, 15;67(6):505-12. Epub 2009 Apr 9.

30. Ramesh B.N., Rao T.S., Prakasam A., Sambamurti K., Rao K.S. (2010). Neuronutrition and Alzheimer's disease. Journal Alzheimers Disease, 19(4),1123-39.

Section V   Disability Awareness

31. Rojas-Fernandez C.H., Moorhouse P. (2009). Current concepts in vascular cognitive impairment and pharmacotherapeutic implications. *Annuals Pharmacotherapy*, 43(7):1310-23. Epub 2009 Jul 7.

32. Rosenthal T., Nussinovitch N. (2008). Managing hypertension in the elderly in light of the changes during aging. *Blood Pressure*, 17(4),186-94.

33. Sanders ,S., Morano, C. (2008). Alzheimer's disease and related dementias. *Journal Gerontological Social Work*, 50 Suppl 1, 191-214.

34. Selhub J., Troen A., Rosenberg I.H. (2010). B vitamins and the aging brain. *Nutrition Review*, 68 Suppl 2, S112-8. doi: 10.1111/j.1753-4887.2010.00346.x.

35. Shagam , J.Y. (2009). The many faces of dementia. *RadiologicalTechnology*, 81(2), 153-68.

36. Shah K., Qureshi S.U., Johnson M., Parikh N., Schulz P.E., Kunik M.E. (2009). Does use of antihypertensive drugs affect the incidence or progression of dementia? A systematic review. *American Journal Geriatric Pharmacotherapy*, 7(5),250-61.

37. Shlyakhto E. (2007). Observational Study on Cognitive function And systolic blood pressure Reduction (OSCAR): preliminary analysis of 6-month data from > 10,000 patients and review of the literature. *Current Medical Research Opinion*, 23 Suppl 5, S13-8.

38. Smith A.D. (2008). The worldwide challenge of the dementias: a role for B vitamins and homocysteine? *Food Nutrition Bulletin*, 29(2 Suppl), S143-72.

39. Solans-Laqué R., Bosch-Gil J.A., Molina-Catenario C.A., Ortega-Aznar A., Alvarez-Sabin J., Vilardell-Tarres M. (2008). Stroke and multi-infarct dementia as presenting symptoms of giant cell arteritis: report of 7 cases and review of the literature. *Medicine* (Baltimore), 87(6),335-44.

40. Sparks D.L., Kryscio R.J., Sabbagh M.N., Connor D.J., Sparks L.M., Liebsack C. (2008). Reduced risk of incident AD with elective statin use in a clinical trial cohort. *Current Alzheimer Research*, 5(4), 416-21.

41. Staekenborg S.S., Su T., van Straaten E.C., Lane R., Scheltens P., Barkhof F., van der Flier W.M. (2010). Behavioural and psychological symptoms in vascular dementia; differences between small- and large-vessel disease. *Journal Neurological Neurosurgical Psychiatry*, 81(5), 547-51. Epub 2009 Dec 3.

42. Teipel S.J., Meindl T., Wagner M., Kohl T., Bürger K., Reiser M.F., Herpertz S., Möller H.J., Hampel H. (2009). White matter microstructure in relation to education in aging and Alzheimer's disease. *Journal Alzheimers Disease*, 17(3),571-83.

43. U.S. Department of Health and Human Services, National Institute on Aging, National Institutes of Health, Alzheimer's Disease Education & Referral Center, NIH Publication No. 08-6423. November 2008 (reprinted February 2010).

44. Vidovich M.R., Lautenschlager N.T., Flicker L., Clare L., Almeida O.P. (2009). The PACE study: a randomised clinical trial of cognitive activity (CA) for older adults with mild cognitive impairment (MCI). *Trials*, 10, 114.

45. Zanetti O, Solerte SB, Cantoni F. (2009). Life expectancy in Alzheimer's disease (AD). *Archives Gerontology Geriatrics*, 49 Suppl 1, 237-43.

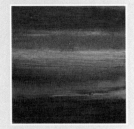

CHAPTER 21

Musculoskeletal Conditions

By Jamie Terry, DPT, CSCS

Jamie Terry, DPT, CSCS,, is a 2010 graduate of the University of Montana School of Physical Therapy.

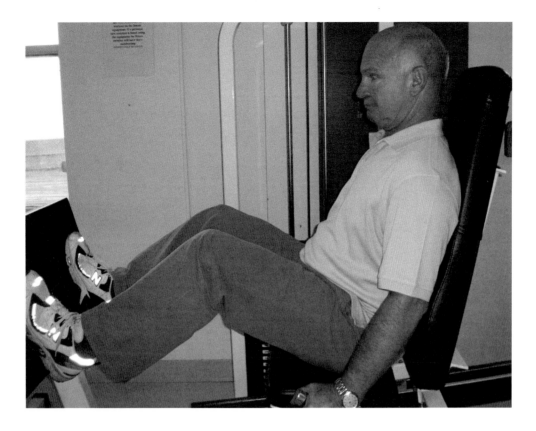

Arthritis

Overview of the Pathophysiology:

Arthridities are a group of conditions involving inflammation and damage to joints of the body. There are over 100 different forms of arthritis, the most common form, osteoarthritis, is a result of repetitive micro-trauma to the joint. Other common forms include rheumatoid arthritis, psoriatic arthritis, lupus and additional autoimmune diseases. Rheumatoid arthritis is a progressive systematic autoimmune disorder presenting with a chronic inflammation of the synovial tissues with periods of exacerbation and remission. Women are three times more likely to be effected and the typical age of onset is between 30 to 50 years of age. Rheumatoid arthritis usually attacks smaller joints such as the joints in the hands or feet and is idiopathic in nature. Osteoarthritis, which is found in the larger joints, has a "wear and tear" etiology. In rheumatoid arthritis the onset of signs and symptoms maybe gradual or immediate and joints affected are usually symmetrical. Classic presentation involves morning stiffness lasting for longer than 30 minutes, warm and painful joints, as well as redness at the joints. Joint deformity, decreased appetite, and fatigue are also present with disease progression.

Medical Management

Arthridities are usually managed conservatively with an emphasis on pain control through exercise, joint protection and pharmaceutical education and administration. Arthridities are multifaceted in nature so medical management should be multidisciplinary involving the primary care physician, pharmacists, and therapists (physical, occupational, recreational) focusing on prevention and rehabilitation. Medications for arthritis are used to control the destructive inflammatory process as well as control pain caused by the chronic inflammation. Current medications work in either a direct or indirect method by controlling the inflammatory response or the autoimmune response (see Table1 below).

Responses to Exercise

Exercise and activity is indicated for these individuals during periods of remission. Weight bearing activity can be performed as tolerated as long as it does not increase the client's pain. Pain levels can be monitored using a visual analog scale (VAS) with levels

Table 1. Arthritis Medications. [1]

Class of Drugs	Purpose	Common Side Effects	Exercise/Activity Cautions
Topical Pain Relievers	Provide quick pain relief for limited effected joints, not severe pain. Common active ingredients are salicylate, capsaicin, or menthol.	Temporary burning or stinging at the site of application	Altered perception of pain
Anti-Inflammatory (NSAIDs) Aspirin, Ibuprofen, Naproxen	Can be over the counter or prescription. Used to relieve swelling, pain and joint stiffness.	Gastrointestinal (GI) distress, ulcers, renal dysfunction Reactions due to prostaglandin production inhibition	Dehydration, altered perception of pain, risk of hyponatremia with endurance activity
Narcotic Pain Relievers	Used for pain relief. Often combined with NSAIDs to enhance their effects. ***Don't mix with acetaminophen (Tylenol) due to risk of liver damage.	Dependence, constipation, drowsiness, dry mouth, and difficultly with urination.	Decreased endurance and activity tolerance
Corticosteroids	Powerful anti-inflammatory	Immune suppression, high blood pressure, bone disease, muscle weakness, weight gain.	Weakened connective tissue (muscles, tendons, ligaments and bones), decreased activity tolerance, increased risk infection secondary to depressed immune function
Disease-Modifying Antirheumatic Drugs (DMARDs)	Alter or suppress immune response. Takes weeks to notice the benefits of taking a DMARD so typically used as second line of defense if NSAIDs don't work.	Nausea, diarrhea, rashes, renal impairment, lung disease, headache, immune suppression.	GI distress, decreased activity tolerance, suppressed immune system

0-10, with 0 being no pain and 10 being worst pain imaginable. During periods of exacerbation bed rest or regular rest periods may be indicated as well as energy conservation techniques, such as breaking up large tasks into small tasks with breaks as needed, and passive range of motion. Hydrotherapy and gentle isometrics will be indicated in subacute stages. Pool exercise, such as water jogging or water aerobics is a great option for individuals with arthritis. The buoyancy of the water will unload the joints while allowing the individual to perform non-weight bearing strength and endurance training.

Special Considerations

Splinting, adaptive equipment, and hydrotherapy are important considerations with this population. Using special adaptive equipment to facilitate hand grasp on workout equipment is important for these individuals. Having an accessible facility and easy access to equipment taking wheelchair adaptability into consideration will be important as well with the progression of the disease.

Osteoporosis

Overview of the Pathophysiology

Osteoporosis is defined as a skeletal disorder characterized by compromised bone strength predisposing a person to an increased risk of fracture.[2] Osteoporosis can be further divided into primary and secondary osteoporosis. Primary osteoporosis can be prevented through achieving maximal peak bone mineral density by the time of physiological maturity. Secondary osteoporosis is a result of medications, other conditions, and/or diseases. To prevent the development of osteoporosis, it is imperative to maintain healthy bone mineral density throughout one's lifespan. A healthy diet and regular exercise are key components toward maintaining healthy bone density. Athletes performing weight-bearing activities tend to have the highest bone mineral density retention. Age is the most important risk factor in the development of osteoporosis. After the fourth decade in life, maintaining bone mineral density is much more difficult due to an imbalance in bone creation and resorbtion. More bone is resorbed into the body than what is created by the body, and this leads to a net loss in bone mineral density.

Osteoporosis can also be a secondary condition for people with diseases or disabilities that affect the amount of weight bearing activity a person is able to perform. Gender is a major risk factor for the development of osteoporosis with females being at greater risk due to lower levels of estrogen in their later years. Younger women are also at greater risk of developing osteoporosis later in life when they develop the "female athlete triad" which consists of patterns of unhealthy eating, excessive exercise, and amenorrhea (absence of menstruation).White women of northwestern European descent appear to have the highest rates of osteoporosis. Environmental factors such as eating habits or dietary restrictions also affect the development of osteoporosis.

Medical Management

Osteoporosis is an asymptomatic condition until a fracture occurs. Individuals who are at risk should be encouraged to take preventative measures by getting their bone density tested and consulting with their primary care physician and pharmacist. With early risk factor identification, nutrition can be adjusted to help manage the disease process. Consultation with a nutritionist will be a key component for the incorporation of a healthy diet to facilitate absorption of supplements as well as medications. See Table 2.

Responses to Exercise

To facilitate optimal bone health exercise and physical activity are highly advocated for this population. There is strong evidence that physical activity early in life contributes to a higher peak bone mass, and it is indicated that resistance and high-impact activity are likely the most beneficial.[3] Once an individual is diagnosed with osteoporosis their exercise program should incorporate both aerobic and strength training activities as well

Table 2. Osteoporosis Medications.[1]

Class of Drugs	Purpose	Common Side Effects	Exercise/Activity Cautions
Calcium Supplements	Adequate calcium for bone formation.	Excessive amounts- Constipation, drowsiness, fatigue, headache	N/A
Vitamin D	Increase absorption and decrease renal excretion of calcium and phosphate.	Excessive amounts- Headache, increased thirst, decreased appetite, metallic taste, fatigue, GI distress.	N/A
Calcitonin	Decreases blood calcium levels and promotes bone mineralization.	Analgesic, GI disturbance, loss of appetite, and redness of the head, hands and feet.	N/A
Bisphosphonates	Reduce bone resorption by inhibiting osteoclast activity.	GI distress, nausea, diarrhea, esophagitis	Possible stomach discomfort during activity
Estrogen	Increase bone mineral content.	Cardiovascular disease, cancer **SERM is alternative with fewer side effects	Moitor cardiovascular response to exercise

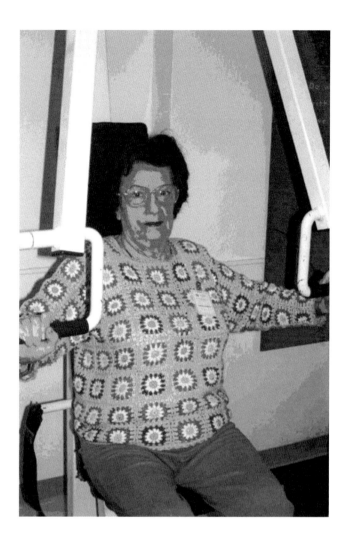

as balance exercises. Strength training should consist of a gentle weight lifting program and yoga or Tai Chi are good options for balance. Always consult with the individual's physician and physical therapist to address safety concerns regarding a specific exercise program.

Special Considerations

Exercise programs for people with osteoporosis should focus on pain free activity and fall prevention. The fear of falling usually outweighs the desire to be physically fit, so these individuals will often stop exercising which ironically increases the risk of falling. Randomized clinical trails of exercise have been shown to reduce the risk of falls by approximately 25%.[2] Make sure clients feels safe and secure while taking part in a fitness program. The Certified Inclusive Fitness Trainer (CIFT) should maintain open communication with the client as well as the client's doctor and nutritionist to ensure proper patient education and disease progression management.

Joint Replacement

Overview of the Pathophysiology

Total joint arthroplasty is a successful and cost-effective procedure for moderate to severe osteoarthritis. The most commonly replaced joints are the knees, hips, and shoulders. There are various surgical approaches for each of these joints. The primary indications for surgery are pain, loss of function, and progression leading towards deformity. Other factors such as motivation, compliance, and support are also taken into consideration when deciding on a potential total joint arthroplasty candidate. A study by Kurtz et al. looked at the prevalence of total knee arthroplasty (TKA) and total hip arthroplasty (THA) and found a steady increase between 1990-2002 particularly in TKAs tripling in numbers and THA increasing by 50%.[4] The rate of revisions for total joints is also increasing in THA and TKA. With these replacement procedures on the rise it is important for the CIFT to have an appreciation for the surgical techniques and to be familiar with contraindications and precautions following surgery. Most of these individuals will not be participating in a training program until they have been discharged from a rehabilitation program; however, post surgical contraindications can persist for years.

Medical Management:

THA is indicated for people who have pain after a long history of osteoarthritis, rheumatoid arthritis, developmental dysplasia, or another pathology compromising the structural integrity and nutrition of the joint. The two main types of THA are cemented and non-cemented. Cemented allows for immediate weight bearing but has a greater

Table 3.

General postoperative precautions: Posterolateral approach	
Avoid hip Adduction	Examples: do not cross legs when sitting or lying down, **DO** use an abduction pillow between the knees while side lying
Avoid hip Medial Rotation	Examples: do not pivot towards surgical side
Avoid hip Flexion >90°	Examples: do not sit on low surfaces, do not lean forward to get up from sitting, do not bend over to tie ones shoes

General postoperative precautions: Anterior approach	
Avoid hip Extension	Examples: do not extend leg behind the body while walking.
Avoid hip Lateral Rotation	Examples: do not pivot away from surgical side while walking and turning or laying and reaching across the body.

propensity for loosening of the prosthesis. A non-cemented prosthesis is toe-touch weight bearing from up to six weeks, but has a longer life expectancy than cemented. Non-cemented also allows a larger amount of bone tissue to remain intact and continued bone growth. See Table 3 for precautions.

TKA is a commonly performed surgical technique for individuals with osteoarthritis or rheumatoid arthritis used to alleviate pain and to improve quality of life. More than 450,000 TKAs are performed a year in the United States and the number is expected double by 2020.[5] Due to this steady increase it is imperative for individuals performing exercise prescription to understand the risk and long-term outcomes of the procedure as well as the contraindications with exercise. There are three basic types of total knee arthroplasties: cementented, non-cemented, and hybrid. The cemented, again like the THA, allows for immediate weight bearing and is generally used for older and sedentary patients. The non-cemented is toe-touch weight bearing for up to six weeks following surgery and has a longer life expectancy than cemented. The femoral, tibial and patellar components are all non-cemented allowing for bone remodeling. The Hybrid is a combination with a cemented tibial component and non-cemented femoral and patellar component. The weight bearing restrictions are similar to non-cemented with toe-touch weight bearing for up to six weeks. The postoperative precautions include maintaining appropriate weight bearing status and post surgical use of knee immobilizer for stability. The patient will be weaned from the immobilizer once they gain "quadriceps control." Prolonged kneeling and jumping should be avoided with these individuals.

TSA is a surgical option for elderly patients who have failed conservative treatments and have cuff-deficient arthritic shoulders. The patient's age, activity level, job requirements, pain and current range of motion will all be taken into consideration when deciding on an appropriate candidate for this surgery.[6] To allow the subscapularis tendon repair to heal, postoperative active strengthening should not begin for six weeks.

Responses to Exercise

Once an individual has achieved an adequate level of strength and function, they will be discharged from surgical precautions and need to develop an exercise program to maintain strength and range of motion. Patients should be encouraged to remain physically active for overall health as well as bone health. There is evidence that increased bone quality will improve fixation and decrease the incidence of early loosening of the prosthesis.[7] Following TKA, quadriceps and hamstring strength have been noted as a primary limiting factor translating into limited functional mobility with activities of daily living such as walking and climbing stairs.[5] Lower extremity weakness and muscular imbalances should be addressed for functional carryover and better outcomes following total joint arthroplasties. Closed chain exercises are recommended for strengthening the muscles of the lower extremities.

Special Considerations

After any type of total joint replacement, the design an exercise program needs to include an assessment of joint loading. wear and tear, and intensity of exercise. While adequate loading is needed to promote bone remodeling, so is joint protection for longevity of the prosthesis. Activities such as swimming, cycling, and light walking enhance cardiovascular endurance with a relatively low load through the joint while maintaining high intensity. Activities such as hiking and jogging increase the force through the joint and should be done at low intensity and with less frequency for better long-term outcomes.

Recommended Readings on Arthritis

- Fitzcharles MA, Lussier D, Shir Y. Management of chronic arthritis pain in the elderly. Drugs and Aging; 27(6):471-90. 2010.
- Gaffo A, Saag KG, Curtis JR. Treatment of rheumatoid arthritis. Am J Health-Syst Pharm 63:2451-2465, 2006.
- Hurkmans E, Van der Giesen FJ, Vliet Vlieland TPM, Schoones J, Van den Ende ECHM. Dynamic exercise programs (aerobic capacity and/or muscle strength training) in patients with rheumatoid arthritis. Cochrane Database of Systematic Reviews 2009.
- Van Den Ende CHM, Vliet Vlieland TPM, Munneke M, and Hazes JMW. Dynamic exercise therapy in rheumatoid arthritis: A systematic review. British Journal of Rheumatology; 37:677-687, 1998.

Recommended Readings on Osteoporosis

- Carter ND, Khan KM, McKay HA, Petit MA, Waterman C, Heinonen A, Janssen PA, Donaldson MG, Mallinson A, Riddell L, Kruse K, Prior JC, Flicker L. Community-based exercise program reduces risk factors for falls in 65-to 75-year-old women with osteoporosis: randomized controlled trial. CMAJ. 167(9):997-1004. 2002.
- Dragoi D, Popescu R, Traistaru R, Matei D, Buzatu AM, Ionovici N, Grecu D. A multidisciplinary approach to patients with femoral neck fracture on an osteoporotic basis. Rom J Morphol Embryol. 2010; 51(4):707-11.
- Homik J, Suarez-Almazor ME, Shea B, Cranney A, Wells GA, Tugwell P. Calcium and vitamin D for corticosteroid-induced osteoporosis. Cochrane Database of Systematic Reviews 2010.
- Smulders E, Weerdesteyn V, Groen BE, Duysens J, Eijsbouts A, Laan R, van Lankveld W. Efficacy of a short multidisciplinary falls prevetion program for elderly persons with osteoporosis and a fall history: a randomized controlled trial. Arch Phys Med Rehabil; 91:1705-11. 2010.
- Rudman D, Kutner MH, Rogers CM, Lubin MF, Fleming GA, Bain RP. Impaired growth hormone secretion in the adult population: Relation to age and adiposity. J Clin Invest. 1991; 77:1361-1369.

Suggested Reading for Joint Replacement

- Minns Lowe CJ, Barker KL, Dewey ME, Sackley CM. Effectiveness of physiotherapy exercise following hip arthroplasty for osteoarthritis: a systematic review of clinical trails. BMC Musculoskelet Disord. 2009 Aug 4;10:98
- Rottinger H. Minimally invasive anterolateral approach for total hip replacement (OCM Technique). Oper Orthop Traumatol. 2010 Oct;22(4):421-30.
- Roy JS, MacDermin JC, Goel D, Faber KJ, Athwal GS, Drosdowech DS. What is a Sucessful Outcome Following Reverse Total Shoulder Arthroplasty? The Open Orthopaedics Journal, 2010;4157-164.
- Santaguida PL, Hawker GA, Hudak PL, Glazier R, Mahomed NN, Kreder HJ, Coyte PC, Wright JG. Patient characteristics affecting the prognosis of total hip and knee joint arthroplasty: a systematic review. Can J Surg. 2008 Dec;51(6):428-36.
- Van de Sande MAJ, Brand R, Rozing PM. Indications, complications, and results of shoulder arthroplasty. Scand J Rheumatol 2006;35:426-434.

References

1. Ciccone, CD (2007). Pharmacology in Rehabilitation: 4th Edition. F.A. Davis Company.

2. Hamdy RC, Broy SB, Morgan SL, Williamson HF. Algorithm for the Management of Osteoporosis. Southern Medical Journal; 103:1009-1015, 2010.

3. NIH Consensus Development Panel on Osteoporosis Prevention, Diagnosis, and Therapy. JAMA Vol 285;785-795, 2001.

4. Kurtz S, Mowat F, Ong K, Chan N, Lau E, Halpern M. Prevalence of primary and revision total hip and knee arthroplasty in the United States from 1990 through 2002. J Bone Joint Surg Am. 2005 Jul;87(7):1487-97.

5. Meier W, Mizner R, Marcus R, Dibble L, Peters C, Lastayo P. Total Knee Arthroplasty: Muscle Impairments, Functional Limitations, and Recommended Rehabilitation Approaches. JOSPT. 2008;38:246-256.

6. Zeman CA, Arcand MA, Cantrell JS, et al: The rotator cuff deficient arthritic shoulder: diagnosis and surgical management. J Am Acad Orthop Surg 6:337-348, 1998.

7. Kuster MS. Exercise recommendations after total joint replacement: a review of the current literature and proposal of scientifically based guidelines. Sports Med. 2002;32(7):433-45.

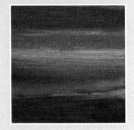

CHAPTER 22

Communication Disorders

By Jessica Malouf, PT, DPT

Jessica Malouf is clinical adjunct faculty at the University of Montana and has also worked in the New Directions Program at the University. She provides physical therapy services and is a staff physical therapist for the Community Bridges Brain Injury Program in Missoula, Mont.

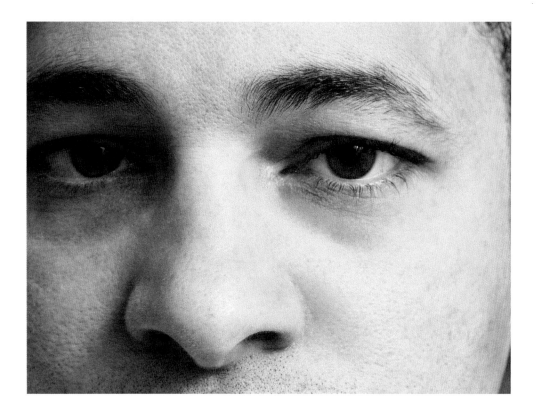

Vision Impairments

Overview

A person has impaired vision if they have difficulty seeing or are unable to see even with the assistance of eyeglasses, contact lenses, medications, or surgery. Vision impairments can be present at birth or acquired in adulthood.

The main causes of vision impairments are age related and include macular degeneration, glaucoma, and cataracts. Other causes of vision impairments include diabetic retinopathy, hypertension, cerebrovascular accident (stroke), atherosclerotic disease in vessels of the eyes, HIV related cytomegalovirus infection, vitamin A deficiency, inflammation of the optic nerve, tumors of the eye, and infections of the eye. Certain medications may also cause vision impairments. Millions of people in the United States have impaired vision.

Regular eye exams can lead to early diagnosis and treatment of eye and vision problems. This is important for maintaining good vision and eye health, and when possible, preventing vision loss. Other ways to prevent impaired vision include smoking cessation; controlling chronic medical conditions through medications, diet, and/or exercise; using UV-protective sunglasses or wide-brimmed hats when in the sun; and using protective eyewear when working with tools or during recreational activities.

Signs and Symptoms

Most vision impairments have a gradual onset. Signs of worsening vision include difficulty seeing objects to either side, difficulty seeing at night or when reading, gradual blurring of vision, difficulty distinguishing colors, blurred vision when trying to view objects near or far, eye itching or discharge, vision changes that seem related to medication.

Treatments

Treatments for vision impairments include low vision devices, medications, and surgical interventions. Examples of low vision devices include spectacle-mounted magnifiers, hand-held or spectacle-mounted telescopes, hand-held and stand magnifiers, and video magnification.

Macular Degeneration Treatments

A higher dietary intake of foods rich in certain carotenoids may lower the risk of developing advanced macular degeneration. One study showed a 43% reduction in risk of developing macular degeneration in individuals with a high intake of dietary carotenoids compared to those with a low intake.[12] Laser photocoagulation is a surgical procedure that is effective in reducing the risk of severe loss of vision and limiting the extent of damage caused by macular degeneration. Although vision, especially central vision, may become severely impaired, complete blindness is not associated with this condition since peripheral vision is usually not affected.

Glaucoma Treatments

Glaucoma is treated with several medications (See Table 1).

Surgical intervention, including laser or incisional techniques, is considered when glaucoma cannot be adequately managed by medical therapy.

Cataract Treatments

Cataract surgery is a common surgical procedure with over 1 million procedures performed annually. Most cataract surgeries today are performed using phacoemulsification techniques. Phacoemulsification involves ultrasonic fragmentation of the lens into fine pieces, which are then aspirated from the eye.

Diabetic Retinopathy Treatment:

Panretinal photocoagulation can reduce the risk of severe vision loss by more than 50 percent if performed early in disease progression. Macular laser therapy can also significantly reduce the risk of visual loss.

Table 1. Typical Glaucoma medications.

Name (actual/ generic) or class	Purpose	Common Side Effects	Exercise/Activity Cautions
Beta-adrenergic antagonists (timolol (Timoptic), levobunolol (Betagan Liquifilm), metipranolol (Optipranolol) and carteolol (Ocupress)	Decrease intraocular pressure by reducing the secretion of aqueous humor by the ciliary body.	Bradycardia, hypotension, heart failure, bronchospasm, syncope, headache, depression, impotence, gastrointestinal disturbance; may mask symptoms of hypoglycemia	Monitor vitals prior to, during, and after exercise. If patient is diabetic, be sure to check blood glucose level before, during, and after exercise as well.
Alpha$_2$-adrenergic agonists (epinephrine (Glaucon), dipivefrin (Propine), apraclonidine (Iodipine) and brimonidine (Alphagan))	Epinephrine and dipivefrin act by increasing conventional and uveoscleral aqueous outflow. Apraclonidine and brimonidine are alpha2 agonists and act by decreasing aqueous secretion.	Headache, sleep disturbance, palpitations, arrhythmia, hypertension, gastrointestinal disturbance, dry mouth, fatigue	Monitor vitals prior to, during, and after exercise. Be sure to monitor heart rate manually instead of with a pulse-oximeter to check for arrhythmia.
Parasympathomimetic agents (pilocarpine (Pilopine HS), Carbachol (Miostat))	Increase aqueous outflow by contraction of the ciliary muscle.	Headache, gastrointestinal disturbance, diaphoresis, dyspnea, bronchospasm, weakness, arrhythmia, hypotension, cholinesterase depletion	Monitor vitals prior to, during, and after exercise. Be sure to monitor heart rate manually instead of with a pulse-oximeter to check for arrhythmia.
Carbonic anhydrase inhibitors (Acetazolamide (Diamox) and methazolamide (Neptazane), dorzolamide (Trusopt) and brinzolamide (Azopt))	Reduce aqueous formation by inhibiting carbonic anhydrase activity in the ciliary body	Taste perversion, anorexia, gastrointestinal disturbance, fatigue, depression, weakness, parasthesias, renal calculi, metabolic acidosis, blood dyscrasias, depressed libido	You may need to adjust the intensity of the workout based on the client's level of fatigue and weakness.
Prostaglandin receptor agonists (latanoprost (Xalatan))	Increases the uveoscleral outflow of aqueous humor	Muscle, joint, back, chest pain; rash	Pain may be a barrier to exercise interventions. Exercises may need to be modified to avoid increased pain. Monitor vitals due to chest pain.

Responses to Exercise

An individual with visual impairment should be able to complete any exercise that a sighted individual can complete as long as the proper assistance is provided. Swimming is a particularly good exercise for those with impaired vision since there are few barriers and a minimal amount of obstacles for the swimmer to avoid. Most pools have lane lines that a client with vision impairment can use to guide them across the pool.

Special Considerations

Initially, the visually impaired individual will most likely require a sighted guide to help them with an exercise program. The fitness professional, as the sighted guide, can provide verbal cueing and physical assistance that will allow the client to safely and comfortably complete an exercise program. Several other device aids that can help assist an individual with vision impairment include (1) the use of a rope connecting one piece of equipment to the next so that the client can guide themselves from one station to the next; (2) large print or Braille on/off switches on the equipment; (3) large print or Braille labels and instructions on the exercise equipment and weights. Certain exercises, like balance and forward bending exercises, may be more uncomfortable and difficult for individuals with impaired vision compared to those with normal vision. Balance exercises are inherently more difficult without the ability to use the visual feedback for postural control and exercises that involve forward bending can create a fear of hitting the head on an unseen object in front of the client. It is also important to consider whether the client's vision impairments are a result of a chronic medical condition, such as diabetes, and to modify the exercise program according to their primary medical condition.

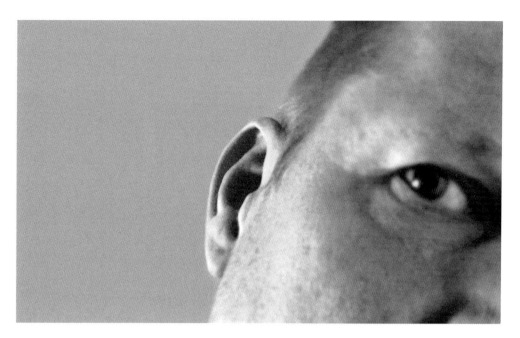

Hearing Impairments

Overview

Hearing impairment refers to both complete and partial loss of the ability to hear. There are three types of hearing impairment: conductive, sensorineural, and mixed. Conductive hearing loss is caused by a problem in the outer or middle ear, such as an infection, and is often medically or surgically treatable. Sensorineural hearing impairment is caused by a problem of the inner ear, or, occasionally with the nerves that supply the inner ear. This type of hearing loss is usually permanent and requires the use of a hearing aid. Sensorineural hearing impairment is commonly caused by excessive noise, aging, and infections such as meningitis, measles rubella and mumps. Mixed hearing loss is when an individual has elements of both conductive and sensorineural hearing impairments.

Hearing impairments can be present at birth or acquired later in life. Causes of hearing loss at birth or early in life include premature birth; lack of oxygen in the womb or during birth; rubella, syphilis or certain other infections in the pregnant mother; inappropriate use of ototoxic drugs (a group of more than 130 drugs, such as the antibiotic gentamicin) during pregnancy; and jaundice in the newborn, which can lead to damage the vestibulochoclear nerve.

Causes of hearing loss later in life include infectious diseases such as meningitis, measles, mumps and chronic ear infections; the use of ototoxic drugs; head injury or injury to the ear; wax or foreign bodies that block the ear canal, and acute and accumulated exposure to excessive noise.

It is estimated that 278 million people in the world have impaired hearing, most of them living in low- and middle-income countries. Many hearing impairments can be prevented with early detection and intervention. Hearing loss can cause delayed language development in children. If hearing is treated and early intervention therapies are accessed, these delays can be minimized.

Signs and Symptoms

Hearing loss can occur suddenly or gradually. Symptoms include inability to hear people clearly and fully, the perception that other people are mumbling, difficulty hearing all parts of a conversation, frequently needing others to repeat or clarify what they have said, reliance on lip reading, fatigue from straining to hear, avoidance of social situations because of difficulty following conversations in noisy environments, and a tendency to pretend to hear others when they really can't.

Treatments

Treatment of hearing loss depends on its cause. Conductive hearing loss is either treated with medication such as antibiotics, or surgery to treat problems with the bones of the inner ear. Sensorineural hearing loss is often treated with hearing aids or cochlear implants. Hearing aids and cochlear implants will not restore normal hearing but they can improve the ability to hear. Aural rehabilitation and auditory training can also be beneficial. This training involves learning good listening strategies and teaching individuals with hearing loss how to set guidelines for communication with others.

Response to Exercise

Individuals with hearing loss will largely have the same response to exercise and gain the same benefits from exercise as individuals with intact hearing.

Special Considerations

Individuals with mild to moderate hearing loss may initially be more successful with their exercise program in a setting with reduced ambient noise. Keeping the radio off or turned down is an easy way to reduce ambient noise. Knowledge of American Sign Language can improve communication ability for a trainer who has clients with hearing impairments, but this is certainly not necessary to create an effective exercise program for these clients. Tools like communication boards can be used to improve efficiency and efficacy of communicating with someone with hearing loss. Figure 1 is an example of suach a communication board.

Figure 1. Communication Board.[13]

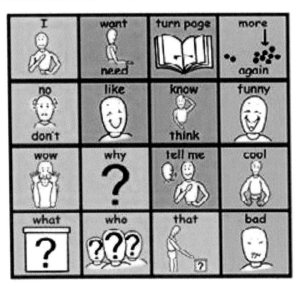

Balance can be impaired with hearing loss if the vestibular apparatus and/or vestibular nerve is affected. It is important to assess and address any balance impairments that may be present with exercise interventions. If the client's hearing loss is caused by a secondary condition that causes developmental disabilities, you may see slower progress with an exercise program than you would in someone with typical development.

People with impaired hearing participate in all types of sports and hearing loss should not preclude anyone from involvement in the sport or exercise program of their choice.

References

1. Acute cytomegalovirus (CMV) infection. Available at: http://www.nlm.nih.gov/medlineplus/ency/article/000568.htm. Accessed January 4, 2012.

2. Lieberman, J.L. Fitness for Individuals who are Visually Impaired, Blind and Deafblind. Available at: http://www.campabilities.org/fitnessactivities.htm. Accessed January 5, 2012.

3. Low Vision Devices. Available at: http://www.aoa.org/x5247.xml. Accessed January 4, 2012.

4. Low Vision Facts - Visual Impairments, Causes, and Treatments. Available at: http://www.lowvisionsolutions.com/resources/visual_impairments.html. Accessed January 4, 2012.

5. Quillen, D.A. Common Causes of Vision Loss in Elderly Patients. Am Fam Physician. 1999 Jul 1; 60(1):99-108. Available at: http://www.aafp.org/afp/1999/0701/p99.html. Accessed January 4, 2012.

6. Torpy, Janet M. Cause of Visual Impairment. JAMA (online). October 15, 2003; 290(15). Available at: http://jama.ama-assn.org/content/290/15/2088.full.pdf. Accessed January 4, 2012.

7. Vision Impairment and Blindness. Available at: http://www.nlm.nih.gov/medlineplus/visionimpairmentandblindness.html. Accessed January 5, 2012.

8. Vision Problems. Available at: http://www.nlm.nih.gov/medlineplus/ency/article/003029.htm. Accessed January 4, 2012.

9. Deafness and hearing impairment. Available at: http://www.who.int/mediacentre/factsheets/fs300/en/index.html. Accessed January 5, 2012.

10. Hearing Loss Signs and Symptoms. Available at: http://www.ucsfhealth.org/conditions/hearing_loss/signs_and_symptoms.html. Accessed January 5, 2012.

11. Hearing Loss Treatment. Available at: http://www.ucsfhealth.org/conditions/hearing_loss/treatment.html. Accessed January 5, 2012.

12. Seddon JM, Ajani UA, Sperduto RD, Hiller R, Blair N, Burton TC, Farber MD, Gragoudas ES, Haller J, Miller DT, et al. Dietary carotenoids, vitamins A, C, and E, and advanced age-related macular degeneration. Eye Disease Case-Control Study Group. JAMA. 1995; 22;273(8):622.

13. Types of AAC used in schools. Available at: https://www.msu.edu/~rbailey/types_of_AAC_used_in_schools.html. Accessed April 11, 2012.

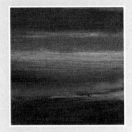

CHAPTER 23

Medical
Disorders

By Yuri Feito, Ph.D., MPH, ACSM-RCEP

and Jessica Malouf, PT, DPT

Dr. Feito is assistant professor of exercise science at Kennesaw State University where he teaches courses in clinical exercise physiology and clinical exercise testing and prescription. He is certified by ACSM as a Registered Clinical Exercise Physiologist and Clinical Exercise Specialist.

Jessica Malouf is clinical adjunct faculty at the University of Montana and has also worked in the New Directions Program at the University. She provides physical therapy services and is a staff physical therapist for the Community Bridges Brain Injury Program in Missoula, Mont.

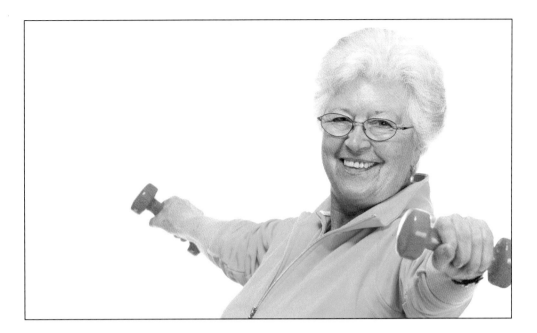

Introduction

Estimates indicate that the population of the United States will be the oldest it has ever been by the year 2030.[16] Improvements in health care and development of preventive health strategies have contributed to increases in life-expectancy over the last century.[16] As the population continues to age, more and more fitness professionals will encounter individuals with at least one chronic condition. The U.S. Center for Disease Control and Prevention (CDC) estimates that by the year 2030, roughly 20% of the U.S. population will be over the age of 65 years[16] and 20% of those will live with at least one chronic condition.[16] Therefore, it is important for fitness professionals to understand how these chronic conditions can affect individuals and how to design exercise prescriptions that are relevant, safe and effective. In this chapter, we will review several medical conditions common to older populations, as well as to others.

Cancer

Overview

Cancer is the general name given to a group of diseases characterized by uncontrolled cell growth resulting from damage to the deoxyribonucleic acid (DNA) of the cell by either internal (*e.g.*, gene mutations) or external factors (*e.g.*, tobacco smoke).[7] Malignant tumors usually grow fast and may spread to other areas of the body (metastasis). Today, millions of people are living with or have experienced cancer, and it is considered the second most common cause of death, behind heart disease, accounting for nearly one in every four deaths.[8] Most cancers are diagnosed in individuals over the age of 55 years;

however, diagnosis can occur at any age.[8] The American Cancer Society estimates that one-third of cancers occurring in 2012 may be prevented with lifestyle changes, such as smoking cessation, limiting time in the sun, being physically active, and eating healthier foods.[8] In addition, the American Cancer Society suggests that screening tests can prevent the development of cancer, improve survival, and decrease mortality by detecting tumors at an early stage when treatment is more effective [9]

Signs & Symptoms

Most early signs and symptoms of cancer are non-specific and may include unexplained weight loss, fever, fatigue, or localized pain.[23] Additional signs and symptoms depend on the type of cancer and are beyond the scope of this chapter. The reader is referred to the American Cancer Society's publication *Cancer: Facts and Figures 2012* for a more detail description of signs and symptoms associated with the specific cancers.[8]

Treatment

The type of cancer diagnosis primarily determines the treatment options. However, three main treatment options exist: surgery, chemotherapy, and radiation therapy.[8]

Surgery: Surgery is the oldest of the treatment options and is the first treatment option for small tumors that have not metastasized (curative surgery). For larger tumors, surgery may be used to reduce the size of the tumor making an individual more susceptible to additional treatment options (*i.e.*, radiation and/or chemotherapy). Side effects may include pain, infection at the site of the wound, pneumonia, bleeding, blood clots, and impaired gastrointestinal (GI) functioning.

Chemotherapy: Chemotherapy refers to the use of drugs to eliminate tumors. Usually, the drugs are given intravenously (IV or into a vein) or taken by mouth. Chemotherapy drugs then travel through the bloodstream reaching cancer cells that may have metastasized. Major side effects of chemotherapy include nausea and vomiting, loss of appetite, hair loss, and mouth sores. Additionally, individuals undergoing chemotherapy are at increased risk of infection (from a shortage of white blood cells), bleeding or bruising after minor cuts or injuries (from reduced blood platelets), and anemia (from low red blood cell counts). Anemia can cause a host of symptoms including fatigue and shortness of breath affecting an individual's ability to exercise and be physical active.

Radiation therapy: Radiation therapy uses high-energy rays (such as x-rays) to remove or shrink the tumor cells. The radiation may come from outside the body, called external radiation, or from radioactive materials placed directly in the tumor (internal or implant radiation). Side effects can include skin irritation and fatigue.

Additional types of cancer treatments include hormone therapy, immunotherapy, targeted therapy, and bone marrow transplantation.[10] The fitness professional should be aware of all treatments and should understand how they affect a person in order to develop safe and effective exercise programs.

Medications

Table 23.1 provides medications along with purpose, common side effects and cautions for exercise for persons with cancer.

Table 23.1. Medications for clients with cancer diagnosis.

Name (actual/ generic) **or class**	**Purpose**	**Common Side Effects**	**Exercise/Activity Cautions**
Chemotherapy (more than 100 different drugs)	• Keep tumor from growing and spreading. • Slow tumor's growth. • Kill tumor cells that may have spread to other parts of the body.	Nausea and vomiting, hair loss, decreased RBC (anemia), decreased WBC (infection), decreased platelet production (bleeding), mouth and throat sores, skin irritation, fertility problems, impaired memory, emotional changes	• Monitor fatigue, shortness of breath and nausea. • Resistance training exercises should be performed on machines instead of free-weights to avoid bruising or potential fractures.
Radiation (external beam and internal implants)	• High dose radiation destroys cancerous cells	Fatigue, skin changes (redness like a sunburn), loss of appetite	Monitor fatigue closely and do not overwork; adjust exercise intensity based on the individual's work ability each day; consider dietitian referral for proper nutritional intake.

RBC = Red Blood Cells; WBC = White Blood Cells

Exercise Testing

When working with individuals undergoing cancer treatment, fitness professionals must consider impairments in functional capacity, musculoskeletal function, and flexibility associated with the disease.[21] For those clients medically cleared to exercise, comprehensive testing to assess body composition, cardiovascular function, musculoskeletal strength and endurance as well as flexibility is appropriate.[7] However, because such comprehensive testing may be difficult for some clients undergoing treatment, those interested in a light intensity exercise program do not require a prior assessment if they have been medically cleared to exercise.[7]

Exercise Prescription

Although specific guidelines for exercise prescription for individuals undergoing cancer treatment do not exist, the American College of Sports Medicine (ACSM) and the American Cancer Society (ACS) recommend and encourage all cancer patient to engage in 30- to 60-minutes of moderate to vigorous intensity physical activity at least 5 days per week.[7] Exercise intensity will vary between clients depending on their treatment and should be closely monitored using VO_2 Reserve (VO_2R), heart rate reserve (HRR), or rate of perceived exertion (RPE). Aerobic exercise should remain moderate [40 to <60% VO2R or HRR or RPE (12-13 in 6-20 scale)] to vigorous [60 to 85% VO_2R or HRR or 14-16 RPE)]. Fitness professionals should be mindful of range of motion limitations when prescribing resistance training (60 to 70% 1-RM) and flexibility exercises.[7] During active cancer treatment short bouts of activity should be encouraged throughout the day, rather than one single session. Once an individual has completed cancer treatment, the exercise session should be developed in the same manner as that for healthy populations, given that the individual does not have any adverse effects to training. [7]

Special Considerations

Consider monitoring the client's fatigue levels before and during an exercise session. Generally every patient undergoing cancer treatment will experience fatigue at some point. If fatigue occurs as a result of the exercise progression, reduce the level without avoiding activity.[7] Start an exercise program with exercises that are well tolerated and progress slowly. Depending on the timing of surgical interventions, the client may have surgical incisions that are healing and/or significant pain upon movement due to surgical trauma. It is important to consider your client's pain when creating the exercise program. Range of motion (ROM) of joints may be affected by scar tissue at the site of surgical intervention as well (*i.e.,* mastectomy scar limiting shoulder ROM). A stretching program is an integral part of any well-rounded exercise program especially when ROM deficits are evident.

Crohn's Disease

Overview

Crohn's disease (CD) is a form of inflammatory bowel disease (IBD) occurring in the digestive track usually affecting the intestines.[20] Crohn's disease can be both painful and debilitating; however, the disease is characterized by a cyclical nature, alternating between active and inactive states.[20] The exact cause of CD is unknown. However as an autoimmune disease, there are treatment options to reduce symptoms, improve quality of life, and minimize short- and long- term toxicity and complications.[18,25] Crohn's disease can occur at any age, but is most likely to develop between the ages of 15 and 35 years.[17] Caucasians have the highest risk of developing the disease but it can affect any ethnic group, and it is usually hereditary. Environmental factors, such as smoking, a family history of the disease and being of Jewish descent may contribute to an increased risk.[25]

Signs and Symptoms

Common signs and symptoms of CD include abdominal cramping/pain, fever, fatigue, reduced appetite and weight loss, pain with passing stool, persistent diarrhea, blood in stool, ulcers in mouth and intestines, fever, fatigue, arthritis, eye inflammation, skin disorders, inflammation of liver or bile ducts, and delayed growth or sexual development in children.[25]

Treatments

A number of treatment options are available to reduce symptoms, improve quality of life and reduce short – and long-term complications.[18] Medications, lifestyle changes and surgery are all appropriate treatment options, depending on the severity of the disease.[17,20,25] Exercise interventions have proven beneficial to reduce symptoms associated with the disease (*e.g.*, bone mineral density; psychological health), although it does not seem to have a direct effect on CD symptoms.[22] Anti-inflammatory drugs, immune system suppressors, antibiotics, and surgery to remove affected portions of the GI tract or scar tissue can also be considered therapeutic options.[25]

Medications

Table 23.2 provides medications along with purpose, common side effects and cautions for exercise for persons with Crohn's disease.

Table 23.2. Medications for clients with Crohn's disease.

Name (actual/ generic) or class	Purpose	Common Side Effects	Exercise/Activity Cautions
Anti-inflammatory drugs (Sulfasalazine, Mesalamine, Corticosteroids)	Reduce inflammation, and reduce symptoms or promote remission of symptoms	Nausea, vomiting, heartburn, headache, diarrhea Corticosteroids: puffy face, excessive facial hair, night sweats, insomnia, hyperactivity, high blood pressure, type 2 diabetes, osteoporosis, bone fractures, cataracts, and an increased susceptibility to infections. Long-term use of corticosteroids in children can lead to stunted growth.	Modify exercises accordingly to improve client comfort. With corticosteroids, use caution with resistance exercises due to effects on bone density, monitor vitals with all exercises, and keep exercise area sanitized due to reduced immune function and increased susceptibility to infections.
Immune system suppressors (Azathioprine (Imuran) and mercaptopurine (Purinethol), Infliximab (Remicade), Adalimumab (Humira), Certolizumab pegol (Cimzia), Methotrexate (Rheumatrex), Cyclosporine (Gengraf, Neoral, Sandimmune), Natalizumab (Tysabri)).	These drugs reduce inflammation by targeting the immune system rather than directly treating inflammation. By suppressing the immune response, inflammation is also reduced since inflammation is an immune system response.	Tuberculosis and other serious infections, increased risk of cancer, serious fungal infections, skin irritation and pain at the injection site (if medication is injectable), nausea, runny nose, upper respiratory infection, headache, abdominal pain, fatigue, scarring of the liver, kidney and liver damage, high blood pressure, seizures, fatal infections, increased risk of lymphoma, multifocal leukoencephalopathy — a brain infection that usually leads to death or severe disability (Natalizumab only)	Modify exercises accordingly to improve client comfort. Monitor vitals with all exercises, and keep exercise area sanitized due to reduced immune function and increased susceptibility to infections. Monitor for signs of liver or kidney dysfunction: frequent urination, yellowing of the skin, significant abdominal weight gain.
Antibiotics (Metronidazole (Flagyl), Ciprofloxacin (Cipro)).	Antibiotics can heal fistulas and abscesses in people with Crohn's disease. Antibiotics help reduce harmful intestinal bacteria and suppress the intestine's immune system.	Numbness and tingling in the hands and feet and, occasionally, muscle pain or weakness, nausea, a metallic taste in the mouth, headache, loss of appetite, vomiting, and tendonitis or tendon rupture (Cipro only).	Monitor for signs of emerging muscle weakness and modify exercises accordingly to prevent soreness. Use caution with resistance exercises or high intensity cardiovascular exercise with clients on Cipro due to possibility of tendonitis and tendon rupture.

Exercise Testing

Exercise testing should be conducted similarly to that of an apparently healthy individual, as long as the individual is not experiencing symptoms associated with the disease. If symptoms are present, exercise testing should be postponed until discomfort decreases.

Exercise Prescription

Current guidelines for CD patients do not exist. However, studies indicate that individuals with CD can benefit from a well-designed exercise program including aerobic and resistance training exercises.[11,20,22] An exercise program will not directly improve symptoms, but can improve comorbidities associated with the disease (*e.g.,* low bone mineral density, quality of life, psychological health).[22] Considering the cyclical nature of the disease, individuals should engage in moderate-to-vigorous intensity exercise during periods when they are not experiencing any symptoms. Overall, medically cleared individuals who are not experiencing symptoms should engage in moderate to vigorous aerobic exercise (40 to 80% VO_2R or HRR) on most days of the week (5 to 7 days/week), and should include resistance training exercises multiple days a week (2 to 3 days/week).

Special Considerations

Dehydration may be common during active states of the disease. Frequent loose stools, excessive drainage, vomiting and/or high body temperature are common symptoms association with CD; thus, fitness professionals should take precautions when an individual is returning to activity to reduce risk of dehydration.[11] The majority of patients develop osteopenia and/or osteoporosis; therefore, fitness professionals should develop exercise programs targeting these conditions.[20]

Diabetes

Overview

Diabetes mellitus (DM) is a metabolic disease characterized by high levels of glucose in the blood stream resulting from a lack of insulin production by the pancreas (type 1); an inability of cells to uptake insulin (type 2); or, a combination of the two.[6] Type 1 DM is caused by an autoimmune response that attacks and destroys the insulin producing cells in the pancreas (*i.e.,* Beta cells). As a result, individuals must use external sources of insulin (*i.e.,* insulin pump or injections).[7] Type 1 DM is not preventable, and accounts for 5-10% of all cases of diabetes. Type 2 DM is the most common (90% of cases) and is characterized by insulin resistance. Insulin is available, however, the target cells (*e.g.,* skeletal muscle, adipose tissue and/or liver cells) are unable to use it, causing high levels of glucose to accumulate in the blood.[6] Another type of DM is gestational diabetes (GDM). Gestational DM occurs during pregnancy, and results in a degree of carbohydrate intolerance of variable severity, causing an increase in blood glucose.[6] Less than

10% of all expecting women experience GDM.[13] Women who develop GDM are at increased risk of developing Type 2 DM later in life.[6]

Signs and Symptoms

The most common criteria for the diagnosis of DM is a fasting blood glucose level $\geq$ 126 mg/dl after an 8 hour fast,[13] However, the measure of glycosylated hemoglobin (HbA$_{1C}$) provides a more accurate estimate of glucose control over several months; therefore, a goal level < 7% is sometimes used as a diagnostic and/or treatment goal.[7] The term "pre-diabetes" is used for those individuals who have levels of blood glucose higher than normal (100 – 125 mg/dl), but cannot be diagnosed as diabetics.[13] Those with pre-diabetes are at a higher risk of developing full-blown diabetes over time.[13]

Some of the typical signs of DM include:[14]

- excessive thirst
- frequent urination
- extreme hunger
- unexplained weight loss
- fatigue
- sudden vision changes
- slow-healing sores
- tingling and numbness in hands or feet
- dry skin
- frequent infections

In addition, nausea, vomiting, or stomach pains may accompany some of these symptoms in the abrupt onset of Type 1 DM.[14]

Treatment

Diabetes treatment requires a lifelong commitment to monitoring blood sugars, healthy eating, exercising regularly, and taking diabetes medication or insulin therapy. For individuals with Type 1 DM, intensive insulin therapy (*e.g.*, injections or via an external pump) is recommended to reduce the risk of short- and long-term related complications (see Box 23.1).[6] For individuals diagnosed with Type 2 DM, the first line of treatment should be the incorporation of lifestyle changes, including increased physical activity and adoption of a heart-healthy diet to achieve a 5% to 10% weight reduction, as the majority of these individuals are overweight and/or obese.[6] Considering the compliance to these lifestyle interventions,[2] most individuals with Type 2 DM eventually require an oral agent, or insulin, to maintain appropriate glucose levels.[6]

According to the American Diabetes Association, diabetes related complications as published on page 145 of *ACSM's Resource Manual for Guidelines for Exercise Testing and Prescription, 6th edition,* include:

- Coronary heart disease death rates in adults with diabetes are two to four times higher than in adults without diabetes.
- Stroke risk is two to four times higher among adults with diabetes.
- Hypertension is present in about 73% of adults with diabetes.

- Retinopathy is the leading cause of new cases of blindness among adults 20 to 74 years old.
- Nephropathy: Diabetes is a leading cause of endstage renal disease, accounting for 43% of new cases.
- Neuropathy: About 65% of people with type 1 or type 2 diabetes have mild to severe forms of nervous system damage involving peripheral motor sensory nerves and autonomic nerves .
- Severe forms of diabetic nerve disease are a major contributing cause of lower-extremity amputations; more than 60% of nontraumatic lower-limb amputations in the United States occur among people with diabetes.

Medications

Table 23.3 provides medications along with purpose, common side effects and cautions for exercise for persons with Diabetes.

Table 23.3. Medications for clients with Diabetes.			
Name (actual/generic) or class	**Purpose**	**Common Side Effects**	**Exercise/Activity Cautions**
Medications that increase insulin production (Dipeptidyl-peptidase 4 (DPP-4) inhibitors: Saxagliptin (Onglyza), Sitagliptin (Januvia); Glucagon-like peptide 1 (GLP-1) agonists: Exenatide (Byetta); Meglitinides: Repaglinide (Prandin), Nateglinide (Starlix); Sulfonylureas: Glipizide (Glucotrol), Glimepiride (Amaryl), Glyburide (DiaBeta, Glynase).	Increase the production of insulin	Upper respiratory tract infection, sore throat, headache; sitagliptin has been associated with severe inflammation of the pancreas, nausea, dizziness, kidney failure (rare), low blood sugar, and weight gain	Keep exercise area sanitized to prevent spreading upper respiratory infections. Monitor dizziness and modify exercises when dizziness is present to reduce falls risk. Monitor blood sugar and modify exercise program accordingly.
Medications that improve the effectiveness of insulin (Metformin: Fortamet, Glucophage, others; Thiazolidinediones: Rosiglitazone (Avandia), Pioglitazone (Actos).		Nausea and diarrhea; rarely, may cause a harmful buildup of lactic acid (lactic acidosis); may cause swelling and weight gain that leads to or worsens heart failure; may increase LDL ("bad") cholesterol; may increase risk of heart attack; rarely, may cause liver problems.	

Exercise Testing

An individual diagnosed with DM is considered a high risk individual per risk-stratification criteria.[7] Careful initial assessment should be performed by appropriate medical personnel. Medical evaluation and exercise testing with electrocardiography is recommended before participation in moderate to vigorous activity.[5]

Exercise Prescription

Exercise is an important tool to support the control of blood sugar, improve overall fitness, and reduce the risk of cardiovascular disease and nerve damage among those with DM. Physical activity and exercise have been shown to be effective in improving insulin sensitivity and facilitate glucose uptake, especially for those with Type 2 DM.[5] However, these benefits are "short-lived" as the effects of an acute bout of exercise lowers blood glucose for 24 to 72 hours.[5] Ongoing participation in physical activity and exercise are paramount for proper glucose control (Table 23.4).

Fitness professionals should design activity programs of moderate intensity (50% to 65% HRR) most days of the week (3-7 days/week) to accumulate 20-60 minutes per session. For individuals who want to participate in more vigorous activities, 65% to 85%

Table 23.4. Effects of Exercise in Diabetes Mellitus[4]		
Parameter	**Type 1**	**Type 2**
Cardiovascular		
Aerobic capacity or fitness level	⇑	⇑/⇔
Resting pulse rate and rate-pressure product	⇓	⇓
RestingBP in mild-moderate hypertensives	⇓	⇓
HR at submaximal loads	⇓	⇓
Lipid and Lipoprotein Alterations		
HDL	⇑	⇑
LDL	⇓/⇔	⇓/⇔
VLDL	⇓	⇓
Total cholesterol	⇔	⇔
Risk ratio (total cholesterol/HDL)	⇓	⇓
Anthropometric Measures		
Body mass	⇓/⇔	⇓
Fat mass, especially in obese persons	⇓	⇓
Fat-free mass	⇑	⇑/⇔
Metabolic Parameters		
Insulin sensitivity and glucose metabolic machinery	⇑	⇑
A_{1c}	⇔	⇓
Postprandial thermogenes is or thermic effect of food	⇑	⇑
Presumed Psychological Outcomes		
Self-concept and self-esteem	⇑	⇑
Depression and anxiety	⇓	⇓
Stress response to psychological stimuli	⇓	⇓

BP, blood pressure; HDL, high-density lipoprotein; HR, heart rate; LDL, low-density lipoprotein; VLDL, very low-density lipoprotein; ↑, increase; ↓, decrease; ⇔, no change. American College of Sports Medicine and American Diabetes Association. Diabetes mellitus and exercise: a joint position statement of the American College of Sports Medicine and the American Diabetes Association. *Med Sci Sport Exerc.* 1997;29:i-vi. American Diabetes Association. Physical activity/exercise and diabetes: position statement. *Diabetes Care.* 2004;27(suppl 1):558-564.

Table 23.5. Practical Recommendations for Exercise for Persons with DM[4]

Perform SBGM	Check before and after each exercise session. Allows the patient to understand glucose response to PA. It is important to ensure that glucose is in relatively good control before beginning exercise. If blood glucose is: >250 mg · dL⁻¹ to 300 mg·dL⁻¹ + ketones, exercise should be postponed. > 250-300 mg · dL⁻¹ without ketones exercise ok, but no vigorous exercise. <100 mg · dL⁻¹, eat a snack consisting of easily absorbed carbohydrates (~20-30 g) 100-240 mg · dL⁻¹, exercise is recommended.
Keep a daily log	Record the time of day the SBGM values are obtained and the amount of any pharmacologic agent (e.g., oral drugs, insulin). Also, approximate the time (min), intensity (HR), and distance (miles or meters) of exercise session. Over time, this aids the patient in understanding the type of glucose response to anticipate from an exercise bout.
Plan for exercise sessions	How much (e.g., time and intensity) exercise is anticipated allows adjusting insulin or oral drugs. If needed, carry extra carbohydrate feedings (~10-15 g · 30 min⁻¹) to limit hypoglycemia. Hydrate before and rehydrate after each exercise session to prevent dehydration.
Modify caloric intake accordingly	Through frequent SBGM, caloric intake can be regulated more carefully on days of and after exercise.
Adjust insulin accordingly	If using insulin, reduce rapid- or short-acting insulin dosage by 50% to limit hypoglycemia episodes.
Exercise with a partner	This affords a support system for the exercise habit. Initially, diabetic patients should exercise with a partner until their glucose response is known.
Wear a diabetes identification tag	A diabetes necklace or shoe tag with relevant medical information should always be worn. Hypoglycemia and other problems can arise that require immediate attention.
Wear good shoes	Always wear proper-fitting and comfortable footwear with socks to minimize foot irritations and limit orthopedic injury to the feet and lower legs.
Practice good hygiene	Always take extra care to inspect feet for any irritation spots to prevent possible infection. Tend to a ll sores immediately, and limit any irritations.

HR, heart rate ; PA, physical activity; SBGM, self-blood glucose monitoring.

©2010 American College of Sports Medicine; and Wolters Kluwer Health; Lippicott, Williams, Wilkins. Used with permission.

Table 23.6. Special Precautions: Recommending Exercise for Patients with Diabetes Complications

COMPLICATION	PRECAUTION
Autonomic neuropathy[α]	Likelihood of hypoglycemia, abnormal BP(⇑/⇓), and impaired thermoregulation. Abnormal resting HR(⇑) and maximal HR (⇓). Impaired SNS or PNS nerves yield abnormal exercise HR, BP, and SV. Use of RPE is suggested. Prone to dehydration and hyper/hypothermia.
Peripheral neuropathy	Avoid exercise that may cause trauma to the feet (e.g., prolonged hiking, jogging, or walking on uneven surfaces). Non-weight-bearing exercises (e.g., cycling, chair exercises, swimming) are most appropriate. Aquatics are not recommended if active ulcers are present. Regular assessment of the feet recommended. Keep feet clean and dry. Choose shoes carefully for proper fit. Avoid activities requiring a great deal of balance.
Nephropathy	Avoid exercise that increases BP (e.g., weight lifting, high-intensity aerobic exercise) and refrain from breath holding. High BP is common. Lower intensity is recommended.
Retinopathy[α, β]	With proliferative and severe stages of retinopathy, avoid vigorous, high-intensity activities that involve breath holding (e.g., weight lifting and isometrics) or overhead lifting. Avoid activities that lower the head (e.g., yoga, gymnastics) or that risk jarring the head. Consult an ophthalmologist for specific restrictions and limitations. In the absence of stress test HR, use of RPE is recommended (10-12 on 20 scale).
Hypertension	Avoid heavy weight lifting or breath holding. Perform dynamic exercises using large muscle groups, such as walking and cycling at a low to moderate intensity.
	Follow BP guidelines. In the absence of stress test HR, use of RPE is recommended (10-12 on 6-20 scale).
All patients	Carry identification with diabetes information.
	Maintain hydration (drink fluids before, during, and after exercise). Avoid exercise in the heat of the day and in direct sunlight (wear hat and sunscreen when in the sun).

BP, blood pressure; HR, heart rate; RPE, rating of perceived exertion; PNS, parasympathetic nervous system; SNS, sympathetic nervous system; SV, stroke volume; ↑, increase; ↓ decrease.
[α]Submaximal exercise testing is recommended for patients with proliferative retinopathy and autonomic neuropathy.
[β]If patient has proliferative retinopathy and has recently undergone photocoagulation or surgical treatment or is not properly treated, exercise is contraindicated.
Reprinted with permission from Campaigne BN, Lampman RL. Exercise in the *Clinical Management of Diabetes Mellitus*. Champaign (IL): Human Kinetics; 1994.

©2010 American College of Sports Medicine; and Wolters Kluwer Health; Lippicott, Williams, Wilkins. Used with permission.

HRR may be prescribed.[5] Resistance and flexibility training programs should be integrated with the aerobic program. Unless the individual has adverse reactions to exercise, the resistance and flexibility prescription recommendations for healthy individuals can be used (2-3 days/week; 8-12 repetitions/set to moderate fatigue; 1-3 sets of 8-12 upper/lower body exercises with a variety of hand-weights, machine weights, bands, free-weights, etc.).[5]

Special Considerations

Considering the glucose lowering effects of exercise, fitness professionals should encourage individuals to monitor blood glucose levels before, during and after an exercise program to avoid hypoglycemia, especially when starting a new exercise program. In addition, individuals taking insulin injections should deliver their insulin dose in nonworking muscles (*e.g.,* stomach) prior to an exercise session. Additional recommendations and precautions are listed in Tables 23.5 and 23.6.

Obesity

Overview

Obesity is a term used for individuals with excessive amounts of body fat. Obesity is a chronic condition believed to be the principal cause of diseases such as heart disease, Type 2 DM, high-blood pressure, and cancer.[15]

Although body fat may be assessed using a variety of methods, the most practical way to determine obesity is revealing an individuals the Body Mass Index (BMI).[1] The BMI is the ratio between body weight and height and is calculated as [weight (kg) / height $(m)^2$].[1] A BMI between 24 – 29.9 kg/m^2 is considered overweight, while a BMI over 30.0 kg/m^2 is considered obese.[1]

Although BMI is a practical measure to determine excess fat, fitness professionals should be aware of the limitations of BMI. Because BMI does not estimate body fat, someone with higher muscle mass may have a high BMI and be considered "overweight and/or obese" while actually lean. Conversely, an individual with a normal BMI may have a high fat percentage and be at risk for cardiovascular and metabolic disease.[1] Because fat distribution has been linked to chronic diseases,[3] another method to estimate body fat distribution may be calculated by using the ratio between a person's waist and hips or Waist-to-Hip ratio (WHR).[3] Standardization of the measurements is critical for an accurate assessment of risk. The fitness professional is referred to the *ACSM Guidelines for Exercise Testing and Prescription* for a detail explanation of these measurements.[7]

Although debate exists as to the "real" cause of obesity, the general assumption is that it occurs due to overconsumption of calories taken in and the lack of enough physical activity (calories in vs. calories out).[7] As such, contributing factors for obesity include physical inactivity, unhealthy eating habits, pregnancy weight gain that is difficult to lose post-pregnancy, poor sleeping habits, certain medications (some antidepressants, anti-seizure medications, diabetes medications, antipsychotic medications, steroids and beta blockers), and medical issues such as Prader-Willi syndrome, Cushing's syndrome, polycystic ovary syndrome, and other diseases and conditions. Some medical problems, such as arthritis, can lead to decreased activity, which may result in weight gain.

Risk factors for obesity include physical inactivity, unhealthy diet, family lifestyle, smoking cessation (may increase appetite), age (activity tends to decrease as we get older), social and economic issues, and certain health conditions as mentioned above. Obesity is linked to conditions such as hyperlipidemia, high blood pressure, type 2 diabetes, metabolic syndrome, heart disease, stroke, cancer, sleep apnea, gall bladder disease, depression, gynecologic problems, non-alcoholic fatty liver, and osteoarthritis.[19]

Signs and Symptoms

Having a BMI over 30.0 kg/m² or a WHR over 0.90 for males and 0.85 for females, is indicative of obesity. Individuals with a BMI of 33 kg/m² have the same risk of cardiovascular death as if they had high blood pressure or high cholesterol.[12]

Treatments

Small changes in weight result in great overall health improvements in obese individuals. Modest weight loss of 5-10% of total body weight have been shown to be target goals to improve health.[7] Lifestyle changes, including dietary restriction and increased physical activity, are paramount for weight loss success, as neither of the two components alone have shown to be effective to combat obesity over the long run.[7] Additional treatment options include the use of behavioral therapies, prescription weight-loss medications, and weight-loss surgery.

Although a detailed nutritional consult with a registered dietitian/nutritionist should be recommended for anyone wishing to establish caloric goals, a safe recommendation is one-to two-pounds of weight loss per week. Individuals should be encouraged to adopt a healthy eating plan including fruits, vegetables, and lean proteins.

Bariatric surgery offers the opportunity for significant losses in body weight; however, this comes at a significant risk. Bariatric surgery may be considered for individuals with BMI greater than 40.0 kg/m², or have a BMI over 35.0 kg/m² along with obesity related conditions (*i.e.,* diabetes or high blood pressure), and have made a commitment to the lifestyle changes necessary for surgery to be successful.[19]

Medications

Table 23.7 provides medications along with purpose, common side effects and cautions for exercise for persons with Obesity.

Exercise Testing

Routine exercise testing is not necessary for individuals with obesity; however, performing an exercise test is recommended to rule out any underlying cardiovascular disease. Additionally, information obtained from an exercise test will aid the fitness professional with the development of the exercise prescription. Although walking is the preferred method for testing, it may not be possible with some individuals and other alternatives should be considered (*e.g.,* recumbent bikes or upper arm ergometers).[19]

Table 23.7. Medications for clients with Obesity.

Name (actual/ generic) or class	Purpose	Common Side Effects	Exercise/Activity Cautions
Prescription Orlistat (Xenical) Non-prescription Alli	Blocks the digestion and absorption of fat in the intestines. FDA approved for adults, adolescents, and children	Oily and frequent bowel movements, bowel urgency, and flatulence with discharge. These side effects can be minimized by reducing fat intake.	Blocks the absorption of some nutrients. Client should take a multivitamin while taking Orlistat to prevent nutritional deficiencies. Client may be fatigued.
Phentermine	Short term weight loss (FDA has approved for 3 months only as it can be habit forming). Appetite reducer.	Dry mouth, unpleasant taste, diarrhea, constipation, vomiting, increased blood pressure, heart palpitations, restlessness, dizziness, tremor, insomnia, shortness of breath, chest pain, dizziness, swelling of the legs and ankles, and difficulty doing exercise that have previously not been difficult.	Side effects such as shortness of breath, dizziness, increased blood pressure, and swelling of the legs and ankles can adversely affect an exercise program.

Exercise Prescription

Obese clients respond well to an appropriately designed exercise program that includes cardiovascular and resistance exercises. However, fitness professionals should be aware of an individual's limitations as he/she may fatigue easily and may have musculoskeletal issues and motivational challenges.

The minimum amount of exercise for weight loss has not been defined;[4] however, evidence suggests any exercise program should include a minimum of 150 minutes per week at a moderate intensity (40% - 60% of VO_2R or HRR) with progression towards vigorous-exercise intensity (60%-80% VO_2R or HRR) to elicit any health benefit.[7] For weight loss and/or maintenance an exercise prescription should include 250-300 minutes per week at a moderate intensity.[7,24] Considering the physical limitations of some of these individuals, physical activity routines may need to be broken down into smaller time increments such as exercise sessions in 10 minute bouts.[7] Promoting physical activity throughout the day, such as using stairs instead of elevators/escalators, parking farther away from a destination, and gardening are additional ways to increase daily activity and promote weight loss.

Resistance training should be part of any well-designed overall exercise program. For individuals with obesity, fitness professional should follow a resistance-training program that engages large muscle groups, at least 2-3 days/week at a moderate intensity (60%-70% 1-RM) for 2 – 4 sets with 8 – 12 repetitions.7 For more deconditioned individuals, one set of 10- to 15-repetitions at moderate intensity is recommended.7

Special Considerations

Development of exercise programs for individuals with obesity should focus on energy expenditure, while reducing the potential for injury.[4] Targeting eating and physical activity behaviors to achieve a energy expenditure goal of 500- to 1000-kcal×day^{-1} is paramount for successful weight loss and management.[7] Considering many obese individuals will have additional comorbidities (*e.g.*, diabetes, cardiovascular disease) the fitness professional is encouraged to perform a comprehensive fitness evaluation prior to designing an exercise program and assess the risk-benefit ratio of starting an exercise program. The fitness professional is encouraged to be aware of additional precautions outlined in other sections of this text or in *ACSM's Guidelines for Exercise Testing and Prescription*[7] depending on the individual's additional comorbidities.

References

1. Clinical guidelines on the identification, evaluation, and treatment of overweight and obesity in adults: executive summary. Expert Panel on the Identification, Evaluation, and Treatment of Overweight in Adults. *The American Journal of Clinical Nutrition.* 1998;68(4):899-917.

2. Intensive blood-glucose control with sulphonylureas or insulin compared with conventional treatment and risk of complications in patients with type 2 diabetes (UKPDS 33). UK Prospective Diabetes Study (UKPDS) Group. *Lancet.* 1998;352(9131):837-53.

3. ACSM. Body Composition Status and Assessment. In: Ehrman JK, ed. *ACSM's Resource Manual for Guidelines for Exercise Testing and Prescription.* Baltimore, MD: Lippincott Williams and Wilkins; 2010. p. 264-81.

4. ACSM. Exercise Prescription for Patients with Comorbidities and Other Chronic Diseases. In: Ehrman JK, ed. *ACSM's Resource Manual for Guidelines for Exercise Testing and Prescription.* Baltimore, MD: Lippincott Williams and Wilkins; 2010. p. 617-34.

5. ACSM. Exercise Prescription in Patients with Diabetes. In: Ehrman JK, ed. *ACSM's Resource Manual for Guidelines for Exercise Testing and Prescription.* Baltimore, MD: Lippincott Williams and Wilkins; 2010. p. 600-16.

6. ACSM. Pathophysiology and Treatment of Metabolic Disease. In: Ehrman JK, ed. *ACSM's Resource Manual for Guidelines for Exercise Testing and Prescription.* Baltimore, MD: Lippincott Williams and Wilkins; 2010. p. 139-49.

7. ACSM. Exercise Prescription For Populations With Other Chronic Diseases And Health Conditions. In: Pescatello LS, ed. *ACSM's Guidelines for Exercise Testing and Prescription.* Baltimore, MD: Lippincott Williams & Wilkins; in Press.

8. American Cancer Society. Cancer Facts and Figures 2010. Atlanta, GA [Accessed July 31, 2012]. Available from: http://www.cancer.org/Research/CancerFactsFigures/CancerFactsFigures/cancer-facts-figures-2012.

9. American Cancer Society. Cancer Prevention & Early Detection Facts & Figures 2012. Atlanta, GA [Accessed July 31, 2012]. Available from: http://www.cancer.org/Research/CancerFactsFigures/CancerPreventionEarlyDetectionFactsFigures/cancer-prevention-early-detection-2012.

10. American Cancer Society. Cancer Treatment and Survivorship Facts & Figures 2012-2013. Atlanta, GA. Available from: http://www.cancer.org/Research/CancerFactsFigures/CancerTreatmentSurvivorshipFactsFigures/index.

11. Ball E. Exercise guidelines for patients with inflammatory bowel disease. *Gastroenterol Nurs.* 1998;21(3):108-11.

12. Bray GA. Obesity: a time bomb to be defused. *Lancet.* 1998;352(9123):160-1.

13. Centers for Disease Control Prevention (CDC). 2011 National Diabetes Fact Sheet. [Accessed July 31, 2012]. Available from: http://www.cdc.gov/diabetes/pubs/general11.htm#what.

14. Centers for Disease Control Prevention (CDC). Basics about diabetes. [Accessed July 31, 2012]. Available from: http://www.cdc.gov/diabetes/consumer/learn.htm.

15. Centers for Disease Control Prevention (CDC). Overweight and Obesity: Causes and Consequences. [Accessed July 31, 2012]. Available from: http://www.cdc.gov/obesity/adult/causes/index.html.

16. Centers for Disease Control Prevention (CDC), The Merck Company Foundation. The State of Aging and Health in America 2007. Whitehouse Station, NJ: The Merck Company Foundation; 2007 [Accessed July 31, 2012]. Available from: www.cdc.gov/aging and www.merck.com/cr.

17. Lichtenstein GR, Hanauer SB, Sandborn WJ. Management of Crohn's disease in adults. The American Journal of gastroenterology. 2009;104(2):465-83; quiz 4, 84.

18. Lichtenstein GR, Yan S, Bala M, Hanauer S. Remission in patients with Crohn's disease is associated with improvement in employment and quality of life and a decrease in hospitalizations and surgeries. The American journal of gastroenterology. 2004;99(1):91-6.

19. Murdy DC, Ehrman JK. Obesity. In: Ehrman JK, ed. Clinical Exercise Physiology. Champaign, IL: Human Kinetics; 2009.

20. Narula N, Fedorak RN. Exercise and inflammatory bowel disease. Can J Gastroenterol. 2008;22(5):497-504.

21. Ness KK, Wall MM, Oakes JM, Robison LL, Gurney JG. Physical performance limitations and participation restrictions among cancer survivors: a population-based study. Annals of epidemiology. 2006;16(3):197-205.

22. Ng V, Millard W, Lebrun C, Howard J. Exercise and Crohn's disease: speculations on potential benefits. Can J Gastroenterol. 2006;20(10):657-60.

23. Schairer JR, Keteyian SJ. Cancer. In: Ehrman JK, Gordon PM, Visich PS, Keteyian SJ, ed. Clinical Exercise Physiology. Champaign, IL: Human Kinetics; 2009. p. 425-42.

24. U.S. Department of Health and Human Services. Physical Activity Guidelines for Americans. 2008 [Accessed July 31, 2012]. Available from: http://www.health.gov/paguidelines/default.aspx.

25. U.S. National Library of Medicine. Cronh's disease. [Accessed July 31, 2012]. Available from: www.ncbi.nlm.nih.gov/pubmedhealth/pmh0001295.

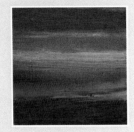

CHAPTER 24

Cardiac & Pulmonary

(obstructive & restrictive)

Disorders

By Brian J. Coyne, M.Ed., RCEP, CIFT

Brian received his Master of Education in Exercise Science from Northeast Louisiana University. He is a Clinical Operations Supervisor in the Cardiac Diagnostic Unit at Duke University Health Systems and has many years of experience in academic, clinical, and wellness settings. Brian has guest lectured, trained graduate students, worked with patients with multiple disorders, and serves as race director for running and triathlon events.

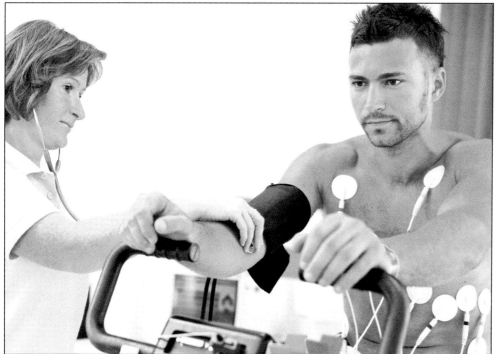

Background

Cardiovascular disease (CVD) is the number one cause of mortality in the United States.[7] Higher rates are seen in people with disabilities or those who have other disorders that limit physical activity. Cardiovascular disease discussions usually focus on coronary artery disease, however cerebrovascular and peripheral arterial diseases are two other forms of cardiovascular disease that have detrimental effects on physical function. CVD also plays a large role in disability determinations and is increased in those with diabetes and other chronic diseases.

Pulmonary disease (PD) – combined numbers for both obstructive and restrictive – is the number three cause of mortality in the United States.[7] PD can cause early functional decrements and be a precursor to cardiovascular disease in those that are at risk of developing cardiovascular disease. The type of pulmonary disease will determine the potential decrement in physical function. The severity of the disease also is a determining factor in one's physical function, just like in cardiovascular disease. Decrements in physical function lead to increases in sedentary lifestyles.

Exercise programming has been used to assist individuals with CVD and/or PD in maintaining, improving, and/or optimizing their physical functioning. Functional limitations, defined by the World Health Organization as any health problem that prevents a person from completing a range of simple and/or complex tasks, can result from limits in physical function as a consequence of both CVD and PD. Individuals with disabilities are at greater risk of developing CVD and/or PD, and statistics show individuals with disabilities have two to three times the rate of CVD as compared to those individuals without disabilities.[5]

Physiology and related science

Cardiovascular diseases cover a wide range of diseases from coronary artery disease, cerebrovascular disease, and peripheral artery disease to obstructive cardiomyopathy. Each of these diseases can produce similar symptoms in the affected areas. For example, peripheral artery disease (PAD) is the buildup of atherosclerotic plaque in the peripheral arteries of the body, while coronary artery disease (CAD) is the same disease process but in the coronary arteries. Both diseases result in claudication (pain resulting from a decrease in blood flow) of the affected areas and subsequently decrease one's physical function. More detailed discussion of the atherosclerotic disease process can be found in the sixth edition of *ACSM's Resource Manual for Guidelines for Exercise Testing and Prescription*.

Other cardiovascular diseases that can affect physical function include, but are not limited to, hypertrophic obstructive cardiomyopathy (HOCM), congestive heart failure (CHF), and ischemic cardiomyopathy. With HOCM the outflow tract is decreased resulting in a decreased stroke volume. To maintain sufficient cardiac output for a set workload, HOCM individuals have a higher heart rate at set workload. With increases in workload as one approaches maximal heart rate, the stroke volume (SV), not peak heart rate (HR), directly relates to peak exercise capacity. The ability of one's heart to fill during diastole allows SV to increase with exercise and helps determine one's peak exercise ability;[6] this is true in persons without disease and patients with HOCM, even though the SV is blunted by obstruction. SV attempts to rise to peak exertion in patients with HOCM, while SV tends to plateau around 40-60% VO_{2max} in sedentary and moderately trained persons without disease. When this occurs in patients with HOCM, sufficient cardiac output cannot be maintained and exercise capacity is limited. Shortness of breath is one symptom typically seen in HOCM patients with exercise. Individuals with HOCM may also have coronary artery disease, but this may not be seen on the 12 lead EKG during exercise due to other EKG changes (*i.e.,* left ventricular hypertrophy, left atrial enlargement) seen at rest in HOCM individuals that make it difficult to interpret changes with exercise. Left ventricular hypertrophy changes (*e.g.,* exaggerated R waves in V5 and V6, exaggerated S waves in V1 and V2, abnormal repolarization represented by T wave inversion and ST segment depression in V5 and V6, left atrial abnormalities, widening of QRS complex), on the 12 lead EKG can mask ischemic changes that may be underlying during exercise.

Individuals with disabilities (*e.g.,* multiple sclerosis, obesity, spinal cord injury, and stroke) can have difficulty thermoregulating body temperature due to their primary disease, and cardiovascular disease can exacerbate this problem, especially in the elderly population. Blood flow to the skin can be decreased in some individuals with cardiovascular disease due to poor shunting of blood to the skin to assist in cooling the body. If this occurs, the core body temperature can reach higher levels and be detrimental to those individuals with disabilities. Individuals with disabilities should take extra preventative measures when exercising in extreme conditions (*e.g.,* heat, cold, at altitude) as they are not as efficient in cooling or heating their own bodies.

Preventative strategies include proper clothing and hydration for exercising in the heat or cold. It is best to use multiple layers of breathable clothing under a windproof shell in the cold. Each layer of clothing will trap air between it, and the body will naturally warm the air held in by the windproof shell. Hot weather clothing should be loose fitting, breathable, and allow moisture to evaporate from the skin. Clothing that "wicks" moisture away from the skin to the outer layer of the garment is best for exercise in warmer temperatures and assists in thermoregulating the body.

Proper hydration is also very important in thermoregulation. Since most exercise bouts for most persons with disabilities do not last longer than one hour, water is the most important element to replenish. These individuals should drink four to eight ounces of water prior to exercise, every 30 minutes during a session, and again afterwards. When an individual is thirsty, they are already dehydrated. One should refer to the ACSM Position Stand on "Exercise and Fluid Replacement" for more information.[4]

Individuals without heart failure are able to pump blood throughout their body at rest and with exercise. Those with heart failure are not able to properly distribute blood as needed, especially to the skin during exercise. Adequate blood flow is required to the skin during higher workloads for cooling of the body during exercise in a warm environment.

Persons with CHF are not able to shunt blood to the working muscles as needed; this is a main reason they cannot obtain high workloads during exercise. Their heart is not able to pump enough blood to the working muscles in response to increases in workloads. This inability to shunt blood as a result of the disease process does not allow them to cool or heat their bodies efficiently. Temperature extremes place a greater demand on their cardiac and pulmonary system as compared to healthy individuals.

Similarly, individuals with pulmonary disease face ventilatory limitations instead of cardiac limitations. As oxygen exchange takes place at the muscle level in the cardiovascular system, oxygen exchange takes place at the alveolar level in the pulmonary system. Obstructive pulmonary disease allows air to reach the alveolar level as it would in a healthy individual. However an individual with obstructive pulmonary disease has a hard time emptying their lungs and allowing proper air exchange to occur. Greater levels of carbon dioxide remain trapped in the lungs; thus less oxygen reaches the alveolar level, which is the area of the lungs where oxygen and carbon dioxide exchange between the lungs and blood takes place. Consequently oxygen is not picked up and carried to the working muscles. This decreased oxygen saturation in the blood means there is less oxygen available for the working muscles to perform work. Lower workloads will be performed at near maximal levels, and a higher heart rate is needed to deliver oxygen to the muscle and compensate for the lower oxygen saturation level. Examples of obstructive pulmonary disease include types of chronic obstructive pulmonary disease (COPD) such as asthma, emphysema, chronic bronchitis.

Individuals with restrictive pulmonary disease face similar challenges in terms of workload limitations. However they are limited by their lungs' ability to inhale sufficient air and oxygen. Restrictive pulmonary disease results in a decreased lung capacity as a result of disease and damage to lung tissue. Decreased viable lung tissue does not allow the lungs to expand sufficiently, thus it takes more effort for these individuals to bring air into their lungs than it does for individuals with non-diseased lungs. This restriction of lung capacity decreases the amount of oxygen reaching the alveoli and working muscles, and limits an individual's work capacity resulting in lower levels of work being performed at peak workloads potentially decreasing the percent of oxygen saturation in the arterial blood, as noninvasively measured by a pulse oximeter. Exercise workloads are limited by the body's ability to take in and deliver oxygen to working muscles and not the body's ability to unload carbon dioxide. Examples of restrictive pulmonary disease include pulmonary fibrosis, asbestosis, and sarcoidosis.

Individuals with disabilities can realize pulmonary limitations as a result of the primary disease process or disability. The pulmonary limitation can be dependent upon their primary disease process, or it can be a comorbidity negatively affecting the primary disease process. Individuals with pulmonary disease as a primary morbidity and those with it as a secondary comorbidity are not able to attain peak workloads as high as those without pulmonary disorders.

Pathophysiology

Decreases in cardiovascular function can result from atherosclerotic or non-atherosclerotic cardiovascular disease or as a result of chronic pulmonary disease. Any of these disease processes can decrease cardiovascular function and subsequent peak exercise capacity. Individuals with congestive heart failure see a reduction in peak exercise capacity. CHF results in a decrease in the heart's function and an increase of fluid in the lungs and/or the periphery depending upon whether the heart failure is systolic or diastolic. Edema in the periphery is a telltale sign of systolic heart failure, while fluid in the lungs can be a sign of either diastolic or systolic heart failure; fluid in the lungs usually occurs after peripheral edema in systolic heart failure. Systolic CHF is a result of damage to the myocardium and a resultant decreased contractility and ejection fraction of the heart. A myocardial infarction (MI) from CAD is one of the main causes of systolic CHF; systolic CHF can develop within hours of an MI. A decreased ejection fraction commonly occurs from systolic cHF. Less force being produced by the left ventricle usually follows, and blood can back up into the periphery and the right side of the heart. Blood will then back up in the lungs. A decrease in systolic blood pressure can also cause blood pooling in the periphery resulting in peripheral edema that is usually seen in the lower legs and feet, hands, and abdomen.

On the other hand, diastolic CHF results from an increased myocardial stiffness when the heart is at rest or relaxed (between heart beats) leading to increased diastolic blood pressure. Long term high blood pressure can cause diastolic CHF. An increased diastolic blood pressure allows less blood to enter the left ventricle between beats. Blood can back up into the lungs and the right heart and venous system, resulting in edema in the lungs and the periphery.

Cardiomyopathies also cause the heart to function improperly and can be associated with CHF as well. Ischemic cardiomyopathy occurs when the heart improperly functions due to ischemia — similar to what happens when there is atherosclerotic plaque in the coronary arteries blocking blood flow and causing inadequate removal of metabolites. Non-ischemic cardiomyopathy is not a result of ischemia but of other origins. For example, hypertrophic obstructive cardiomyopathy is due to long-standing hypertension and can decrease the outflow tract and the heart's stroke volume – amount of blood pumped with each beat. Both ischemic and non-ischemic cardiomyopathy can result in decreased functional capacity and poor quality of life if not treated properly.

Functional capacity decreases in part due to decreased vascular perfusion of the muscles as a result of increased blood pressure or a reduced ejection fraction. A resultant decrease in muscular function occurs from a decreased delivery of nutrients and clearance of waste products. Muscle atrophy has also been shown to occur over time – whether it is from the aging process, the disease process, or a combination of both is yet to be determined.

Pulmonary diseases, like cardiac diseases, can be divided into obstructive and restrictive diseases. Obstructive pulmonary diseases include asthma, chronic obstructive pulmonary disease (COPD), and emphysema. Asthma is typically caused by genetic and environmental factors, results in a restriction of bronchioles from bronchospasms, and is reversible with medication. Smoking is the main cause of COPD, which results in small-airway obstruction, and is not reversible. Emphysema also can be caused by smoking and results in small-airway obstruction, specifically destruction of alveoli sacs, and is not reversible.

Individuals with obstructive pulmonary disease see a reduction in the amount of air they can maximally expire in 1 second (FEV1/FVC ratio) but have a normal forced vital capacity (FVC) — the total amount of air they can expire after a maximal inhalation. Due to the obstructive pulmonary disease, it takes the lungs longer to expire the air inside the lungs after a maximal inspiration. Individuals with severe COPD can have a reduced FVC with a large increase in residual volume due to a large amount of air trapping; this air trapping occurs in the small airways.

Restrictive pulmonary diseases, on the other hand, do not affect the FEV1/FVC ratio. Individuals with restrictive pulmonary disease have a limited FVC and typically a normal or elevated FEV1/FVC ratio; they cannot inspire as much as a "healthy" individual of the same age, gender, height, and race as themselves. Pulmonary fibrosis, asbestosis, and sarcoidosis are a few restrictive pulmonary diseases that result in a decreased lung volume and an increased work to breathe. FEV1 is usually reduced with restrictive pulmonary disease as well; this is why the FEV1/FVC ratio is typically normal or even elevated.

Health Appraisal, Fitness Assessment, and Clinical Exercise Testing

Components of the health appraisal and fitness assessment for persons with disabilities are similar to those without disabilities. The Physical Activity Readiness Questionnaire (PAR-Q) is recommended for individuals without disabilities to screen individual's readiness to exercise. This questionnaire can also be used to assess exercise readiness for individuals with disabilities when they choose to start an exercise program without the referral of a physician. If used properly, the PAR-Q can help provide a risk stratification for an individual so that they can be identified as someone who needs to see a physician prior to starting an exercise program, and/or secure a physician's clearance at a minimum.

Once an individual has been cleared to exercise either through the PAR-Q or their physician, a health history questionnaire can be completed in cooperation with the individual. ACSM risk stratification guidelines for known cardiac, pulmonary, and/or metabolic disease should also be followed.[2] Even though the PAR-Q includes a question about physical activity, it is best to assess physical activity habits either by including questions on the health history questionnaire or by using another tool. Activity questionnaires are a helpful way to determine an individual's recent physical activity history. Some activity questionnaires include the Duke Activity Score Index (DASI), the Stanford Physical Activity Questionnaire, the International Physical Activity Questionnaire (IPAQ), the Physical Activity Scale for the Elderly (PASE), and the Daily Activity Questionnaire in Heart Failure (DAQIHF). Activity questionnaires can be used to estimate daily energy expenditure and/or predict VO_{2peak} in individuals with disabilities.

Even though some of the questionnaires listed above (*i.e.,* Stanford Physical Activity Questionnaire, IPAQ, and PASE) were developed for use with people without disabilities they can still be used to estimate the energy expenditure or physical activity of people with disabilities, if used as a serial comparison in individual clients. The DAQIHF is specific to the heart failure population, but again it could be used by persons with disabilities if used as a serial comparison in individual clients. The DASI was developed to be used over a wider range of individuals to estimate VO_{2peak} based on the activities one is able to complete.

Other questionnaires can also be used to subjectively measure quality of life (*e.g.,* SF-36) or mental health status (*e.g.,* Beck Depression Index). Individual quality of life usually refers to one's general well-being and their ability to perform ADLs, complete more advanced activities, and satisfaction with life. These questionnaires are helpful when determining readiness to exercise as well as emotional health. They can also be given to individuals with disabilities to monitor progress during an exercise program. Two benefits of an exercise program are improved quality of life and increased self-confidence. Serial questionnaires should show improvement in the quality of life and mental health status.

Considerations and modifications to the fitness assessments being completed may need to be made, depending on the severity of disease. The fitness professional must understand how to modify a fitness assessment and testing to fit a person with cardiopulmonary disorders. These modifications could include equipment, protocol selection, or order of assessments. The recommended order of assessment by ACSM is resting measurements, body composition, cardiovascular assessment, muscular fitness assessment, and flexibility assessment.[2] To obtain accurate results for each assessment in individuals with disabilities, the testing may need to be completed on different days. Fitness professionals assessing individuals with disabilities must also be familiar with the absolute and relative contraindications to exercise testing as published by the ACSM and American Heart Association.[2]

Functional assessments are another tool to assess functional fitness levels in addition to clinical cardiovascular assessments. Cardiovascular functional assessments are submaximal evaluations that can be performed on individuals who are not predicted to reach sufficient workloads during cardiopulmonary testing. The six minute walk is a common functional assessment used to measure functional capacity. Fitness professionals should refer to the 2002 American Thoracic Society (ATS) for guidelines regarding administration of the *Six Minute Walk Test.*[21] CHF and COPD client mortality rates have been shown to relate to six minute walk distances. Persons with cardiovascular and/or pulmonary disorders have lower six minute walk distances and have higher mortality rates.[14] The two minute walk-in-place test has been used with individuals unable to walk for 6 minutes[12] and results correlate with disease severity; those with low two minute walk test results typically have higher severity of disease and a higher mortality rate. Individuals who use a wheelchair and individuals with cardiopulmonary disorders with limited mobility can use an arm crank or upper body ergometer to assess cardiovascular fitness.

Muscular strength and/or endurance testing should be done with individuals who have cardiopulmonary disorders. Various tests can be performed and should be joint specific. To assess an individual's lower body endurance, the practitioner could have their client complete the 30 second sit-to-stand test.[16] The arm curl test[12] can be used to assess upper body muscular endurance, even though it is specific to the endurance of the elbow flexors. Since these muscles are used during a multitude of ADLs, it is a good assessment to complete in individuals with disabilities.

Muscular strength testing (*i.e.,* 1-RM testing) can be done in this population, but it should be done with caution – for example in individuals with severe pulmonary disease whose risk would outweigh the benefit of testing. Estimates of 1-RM can be calculated from submaximal testing. The ACSM equation can be used to estimate 1-RM.[2] One RM testing should be joint specific and be of value to the exercise plan before being administered. Other RM (1, 5, 10 reps) equations can be found in the National Strength and Conditioning Association's *Essential of Strength Training and Conditioning*[8]

Flexibility assessment should be done at all major joints and specifically at any joint affected by the disease process. Flexibility is joint dependent and depends on joint structure, ligaments, muscle, and tendons around the joint. Goniometry, a direct measurement of flexibility, should be performed at all major joints and any affected by the specific disease process.

Indirect measurements of flexibility can be done as well and include multiple joints working in concert together. Examples include the upper body stretch (also known as the Back Scratch test or "zipper stretch") and the chair sit and reach test to assess low back and hamstring flexibility. Individuals who score higher in these assessments usually are able to complete ADLs with less risk of joint or muscle injury due to lack of flexibility.[9]

Agility testing is also useful to assess an individual's potential to complete ADLs with little fatigue. The Get Up and Go test is a common assessment used. The test measures the distance covered in 8 seconds from a seated position in a chair to standing and walking forward. Those covering a greater distance have been found to complete ADLs with greater ease.[17] It is also valuable in assessing those at risk for falls since the distance covered in 8 seconds may correlate to one's ability to ambulate without falling.[10]

Each of the above assessment components should be done serially to monitor the response of individuals with cardiopulmonary disorders with regard to the exercise program or treatment plan. The same assessments should be completed at least pre- and post-exercise training or treatment plan; typically four to eight weeks is sufficient time to see improvement in flexibility. Clinical decisions can be made based on the assessment results. An individual's functional capabilities can also be used to predict mortality rates as compared to norms.[11]

Individuals with cardiopulmonary disorders have different responses to exercise as compared to those individuals without cardiopulmonary disorders. These include higher resting heart and respiratory rates and faster increases in HR and respiratory response to the same workload. Blood pressure may see an exaggerated response due to a lack of vascular space for normal blood flow. These responses result in a reduced VO_{2peak} and an increased need for VO_2 at submaximal workloads – resulting from a higher heart rate and respiratory rate at submaximal workloads in addition to the inability to potentially oxygenate and deliver blood to working tissue.

Exercise Prescription and Programming, Safety of Testing and Training

The goals of an exercise training program should be to make activities of daily living (ADLs) "easier" and promote a higher level of wellness for the individual with cardiopulmonary disorders. Exercise trained individuals will be able to complete activities (ADLs and exercise) at lower levels of their maximal functional capacity resulting in fewer metabolites (*e.g.*, CO_2, lactate + H+) being produced and less fatigue. They may also realize an increase in the submaximal workload they are able to achieve – similar to individuals without disabilities – even if they do not increase their maximal functional capacity.

Benefits of exercise training are many. Exercise training has been shown to improve vascular function in those with and without cardiovascular disease.[19, 24] Both aerobic and resistance training studies have shown beneficial effects.

Cardiovascular training helps the working muscles extract more oxygen from the blood received and work more efficiently with less oxygen at set workloads. Individuals with CVD and/or PD will realize similar benefits to exercise training as those without disease; however, they may not see the same percentage increase in functional capacity due to disease limitations. Those with disease can still increase their submaximal work capacity and perform their daily tasks and physical activity at lower levels of their maximal functional capacity. This will result in less fatigue and fewer metabolites being produced during the activity.

Resistance training is also important for individuals with disabilities. The benefits of resistance training seen in individuals with disabilities are mainly the same as those seen in individuals without disabilities – refer to *ACSM's Resource Manual for Guidlines for Exercise Testing and Prescription*[1] for generalized benefits. Resistance training also helps decrease vascular resistance and improves peripheral blood flow resulting in more nutrients reaching the active muscles.[19] More work can then be performed resulting in greater near maximal workloads being achieved and greater muscle strength and/or endurance being realized through training.

Flexibility training is necessary to maintain joint-specific range of motion. Specific exercises should be done at all major joints to maintain and potentially increase range of motion where appropriate. The goal of flexibility training in joints limited by specific disabilities should be to maintain range of motion in the connective tissue surrounding the joint. In those joints not limited by disability or disease, the goal should be to increase range of motion. Increasing flexibility allows joints to work in movement-specific ranges of motion with less risk of injury.

Modifications in the exercise program for the individual with cardiopulmonary disorders may need to be made based on the disease process – Table 24.1 includes brief details for each disease state; for specifics see *ACSM's Exercise Management for Persons with Chronic Diseases and Disabilities*.[3] Various modes of exercise can be adapted to meet the

TABLE 24.1: Exercise programming modifications based on cardiopulmonary disorder

Disorder	Mode of Exercise	Goals	Intensity	Frequency	Duration
Coronary Artery Disease	• Large muscle activity, arm ergometry • Circuit training – major muscle groups	• Increase aerobic capacity • Increase muscle strength and endurance	• RPE 11-16/20; 40-80% HR reserve or VO2max • 30-60% 1RM	• > 3 days/week • 2-3 days/week	• 20-60 min./session • 8-10 exercises; 1-3 sets of 12-15 reps
Peripheral Artery Disease	• Large muscle groups; walking optimal	• Improve walking time before claudication pain • Increase ability to perform ADLs	• 40-60% HR reserve or VO2max • Resistance able to lift 10 times	• 3-5 days/week • 2-3 days/week	• 15-60 min. • 8-12 exercises; 1-3 sets of 10-15 reps
Hypertrophic Obstructive Cardiomyopathy	• Large muscle groups • Circuit training	• Decrease BP at rest and during exercise • Increase muscle endurance and strength	• 40-60% HR reserve or VO2max • 50-80% of 1RM	• 4-7 days/week • 2-3 days/week	• 30-60 min. • 8-12 exercises; 1-3 sets; 8-12 reps
Congestive Heart Failure	• Large muscle groups • Circuit training	• Increase peak endurance capacity • Increase strength; reduce muscle atrophy	• RPE 11-14/20; 40-70% HR reserve or VO2max • Low resistance	• 4-7 days/week • 3 days/week	• 20-60 min./day • 8-10 exercises; 1-3 sets; 10-15 reps
Ischemic Cardiomyopathy	• Large muscle activity • Circuit training – major muscle groups	• Increase aerobic capacity • Increase muscle strength and endurance	• RPE 11-16/20; 40-80% HR reserve or VO2max • 30-60% 1RM	• > 3 days/week • 2-3 days/week	• 20-40 min./session • 8-10 exercises; 1-3 sets of 12-15 reps
Chronic Obstructive Pulmonary Disease, Asthma, & Emphysema	• Large muscle activity • Isotonic machines or free weights	• Increase time to dyspnea • Increase strength	• RPE 11-13/20 • Low resistance	• 3-5 days/week • 2-3 days/week	• 15-30 min./day • 8-10 exercises; 1-3 sets of 12-15 reps
Chronic Restrictive Pulmonary Disease	• Large muscle activity • Isotonic machines or free weights	• Increase time to dyspnea • Increase strength	• RPE 11-13/20 • Low resistance	• 3-5 days/week • 2-3 days/week	• 20-60 min./day • 8-10 exercises; 1-3 set; 12-15 reps

Adapted from *ACSM's Exercise Management for Persons with Chronic Diseases and Disabilities*, 3rd edition, 2009.

needs of individuals with disabilities. For example, many treadmills have side handrails which assist with balance. Seated or recumbent exercise may also be less strenuous for individuals with disabilities since the body is supported during exercise thus lowering the needed VO_2 during exercise. Resistance exercises can also be adapted to meet the needs of individuals with disabilities.

For example, cardiovascular training programs can use short bouts of exercise to elicit the expected cardiovascular benefits discussed in this chapter. The intensity of exercise can be higher during the short bouts than would be achieved during longer duration. Duration can be maintained at recommended levels (30 minutes of moderate intensity or 20 minutes of vigorous intensity) with short bouts followed by brief rest periods.

The prescribed frequency and duration of exercise for an individual with cardiopulmonary disorders should be similar to an individual without disabilities, however the intensity will be lower — see *ACSM's Guidelines for Exercise Testing and Prescription* for more information for recommendations.[2] The duration and intensity of individual exercise bouts can be modified as needed based on heart rate, blood pressure, respiratory rate, and ratings of perceived exertion. Medications (*e.g.,* beta-blockers) can dampen one's response to the duration and intensity of exercise, specifically heart rate and blood pressure. Medications may also have a beneficial response to the exercise capacity. For more information regarding a summary of heart rate, blood pressures, and exercise capacity responses to exercise, see "Appendix B" in *ACSM's Guidelines for Exercise Testing and Prescription, Eighth Edition.*[2]

Heart rate responses and other measures of exertion in persons with cardiovascular and/or pulmonary disorders should be monitored throughout each exercise session. Heart rate can be monitored with a heart rate monitor, if available, or palpation. The rating of perceived exertion (RPE) scale is also a useful method to monitor the client's response to

Table 24.2: Modified Borg RPE scale

0	Nothing at all
0.5	Extremely weak
1	Very weak
2	Weak
3	Moderate
4	
5	Strong
6	
7	Very Strong
8	
9	Extremely Strong
10	

Adapted from Borg, G., *Borg's Perceived Exertion and Pain Scales.* Champaign, IL: Human Kinetics; 1998.

Table 24.3: Symptom scale (pain scale)

0	zNone
0.5	Just noticeable
1	
2	Light
3	
4	
5	Heavy
6	
7	
8	
9	Maximum pain
10	

Adapted from Borg, G., *Borg's Perceived Exertion and Pain Scales.* Champaign, IL: Human Kinetics; 1998.

exercise. Another useful method to monitor subjective exercise intensity, the modified Borg RPE scale (Table 24.2), is effective in evaluating the client's response to exercise. It can also be used as a "symptom scale" (Table 24.3), specifically to measure an individual's chest pain, dyspnea or shortness of breath, or other symptom. It is expected that individuals with cardiovascular and/or pulmonary disorders will have similar responses to those without disorders, however the workloads attained and progression of exercise will be lower on average in those with disorders. The dyspnea scale (Table24.4) can be used to monitor shortness of breath in individuals with pulmonary disease.[23]

Individuals with cardiovascular and/or pulmonary disorders also need to adhere to the prescribed medication regimen. Taking medications regularly and at similar times of day should help to improve the client's ability to exercise. Medications prescribed for an individual with cardiovascular and/or pulmonary limitations are meant to decrease the workload of the cardiac and/or pulmonary system(s) and make life easier for those individuals. For example, beta-blockers taken for high blood pressure assist in decreasing the

Table 24.4: Dyspnea scale

0	No trouble breathing
1	Short of breath hurrying on level ground or walking up slight uphill
2	Have to stop when walking at own pace on level ground
3	Short of breath and stops after walking approximately 100 meters
4	Unable to leave house due to breathlessness

Adapted from Doherty, D.E. et al. Chronic Obstructive Pulmonary Disease: Consensus Recommendations for Early Diagnosis and Treatment, *The Journal of Family Practice,* S1-S8, 2006.

heart's workload. They decrease the heart rate and allow the heart to fill with more blood between beats, thus maintaining stroke volume and cardiac output.

Modifications to cardiovascular assessment or training may be made for those unable to perform lower body cardiovascular exercise with safety. For those individuals, the fitness professional should expect heart rate and blood responses to be higher at absolute workloads as compared to lower body exercise. Upper body exercise elicits a higher heart rate and blood pressure as compared to lower body exercise; a smaller muscle mass is used during upper body exercise. Thus one cannot perform upper body exercise at the same absolute workload lower body exercise would be completed with. Either the duration must be shortened or the intensity can be decreased so exercise can last longer at a reduced workload. Once the individual becomes accustomed to upper body exercise, the duration can be increased followed by the intensity. Fitness professionals need to select appropriate exercise modalities for individuals with disabilities and need to know how to modify exercises to fit the needs of the clients. Safety is a major concern and can help prevent injuries. Injury can limit exercise training and adversely affect functional capacity in persons with cardiopulmonary disorders.

Summary

Exercise is important and aids individuals with cardiovascular and/or pulmonary disease in maintaining and/or improving their functional ability while helping to decrease the risk for future cardiac and/or pulmonary events. Assessing the functional capacity of individuals with cardiovascular and/or pulmonary disease allows medical care providers to make clinical decisions that helps to improve the client's clinical status. Fitness professionals play a vital role in assisting individuals with cardiovascular and/or pulmonary disease and help them to maintain and/or improve overall health. Exercise training, medication compliance, and other lifestyle modifications allow individuals with cardiovascular and/or pulmonary disease to live fruitful lives.

Additional Resources

Note to Reader: For a more detailed discussion on any of these cardiopulmonary disorders, there are multiple sources available. Some include the following and are useful reference materials:

- *Pollock's Textbook of Cardiovascular Disease and Rehabilitation* edited by J.L. Durstine, G.E. Moor, M.J. LaMonte, and B.A. Franklin – Human Kinetics publisher
- *Clinical Exercise Physiology* edited by J. Ehrman, S. Keteyian, P., & P. Visich – Human Kinetics publisher
- *ACSM's Resources for the Clinical Exercise Physiologist* – Lippincott Williams & Wilkins publisher

References

1. American College of Sports Medicine. *ACSM's Resource Manual for the Guidelines for Exercise Testing and Prescription*, 6th Ed. Lippincott, Williams, & Wilkins, Baltimore, MD, 2009.

2. American College of Sports Medicine. *ACSM's Guidelines for Exercise Testing and Prescription*, 8th ed. Lippincott, Williams, & Wilkins, Baltimore, MD, 2009.

3. American College of Sports Medicine. *ACSM's Exercise Management for Persons with Chronic Diseases and Disabilities*, 3rd ed., Human Kinetics: Chicago, IL, 2009.

4. American College of Sports Medicine. ACSM Position Stand: Exercise and Fluid Replacement, *Med Sci Sports Exerc*, 1996.

5. Centers for Disease Control and Prevention (CDC). *Behavioral Risk Factor Surveillance System Survey Data*. Atlanta, Georgia: U.S. Department of Health and Human Services, Centers for Disease Control and Prevention, 2010.

6. Lele, S.S., Thomson, H.L., Seo, H., Belenkie, I., McKenna, W.J., & Frenneaux, M.P. Exercise Capacity in Hypertrophic Cardiomyopathy: Role of Stroke Volume Limitation, Heart Rate, and Diastolic Filling Characteristics, *Circulation*, 92:2886-2894, 1995.

7. National Center for Health Statistics. Health, United States, 2010: With Special Feature on Death and Dying. Hyattsville, Maryland. 2011.

8. National Strength and Conditioning Association. *Essential of Strength Training and Conditioning*, T.R. Baechle, editor, 3rd edition, 2008.

9. Olivares PR, Gusi N, Prieto J, & Hernandez-Mocholi MA, Fitness and health-related quality of life dimensions in community-dwelling middle aged and older adults, *Health Qual Life Outcomes*, Dec 22; 9:117, 2011.

10. Beauchet O, Fantino B, Allali G, Muir SW, Montero-Odasso M, Annweiler C, Timed Up and Go test and risk of falls in older adults: a systematic review, *J Nutr Health Aging*, 15(10):933-8, 2011.

11. Tsiouris A, Horst HM, Paone G, Hodari A, Eichenhorn M, Rubinfeld I. Preoperative risk stratification for thoracic surgery using the American College of Surgeons National Surgical Quality Improvement Program data set: Functional status predicts morbidity and mortality. *J Surg Res.*, 2012 Mar 13.

12. Jones C.J., & Rikli R.E., Measuring functional fitness of older adults, *The Journal on Active Aging*, March April 2002, pp. 24–30.

13. Ró a ska-Kirschke, A., Kocur, P., Wilk, M., Dylewicz, P., The Fullerton Fitness Test as an index of fitness in the elderly. *Medical Rehabilitation* 2006; 10(2): 9-16.

14. Boxer, R., Kleppinger, A., Ahmad, A., Annis, K., Hager, D., & Kenny, A. The 6-Minute Walk is Associated With Frailty and Predicts Mortality in Older Adults With Heart Failure, *Congestive Heart Failure*, 2010: 16:208-213.

15. Rikli, R.E. & Jones, C.J. *Senior Fitness Test Manual*. Human Kinetics, Chicago, IL, 2001.

16. Jones, CJ, Rikli RE, Beam WC. A 30-s chair-stand test as a measure of lower body strength in community-residing older adults. *Research Quarterly for Exercise and Sport*. 1999;70:113-119.

17. Mathias S, Nayak USL, Isaacs B. Balance in elderly patients: the "get-up and go" test. *Arch Phys Med Rehabil*. 1986;67:387-389.

18. Rostagno C, Olivo G, Comeglio M, Boddi V, Banchelli M, Galanti G, Gensini GF. Prognostic value of 6-minute walk corridor test in patients with mild to moderate heart failure: comparison with other methods of functional evaluation. *European Journal of Heart Failure* (2003) Jun; 5(3): 247-52.

19. Dobrosielski, D.A., Greenway, F., Welsh, D.A., Jazwinski, S.M., & M. A. Welsch. Modification of Vascular Function following Handgrip Exercise Training in 73-90 year Old Men. *Medicine and Science in Sports and Exercise*, 2009.

20. Garet M, Barthelemy JC, Degache F, Costes F, Da-Costa A, Isaaz K, Lacour JR, Roche F. A questionnaire-based assessment of daily physical activity in heart failure. *European Journal of Heart Failure* (2004) Aug;6(5):577-84.

21. American Thoracic Society statement: guidelines for the six-minute walk test. ATS Committee on Proficiency Standards for Clinical Pulmonary Function Laboratories. *Am J Respir Crit Care Med* 2002;166(1):111-117.

22. Borg, G., Borg's Perceived Exertion and Pain Scales. Champaign, IL: Human Kinetics; 1998.

23. Doherty, D.E., Belfer, M.H., Brunton, S.A., Fromer, L., Morris, C.M., Snader, T.C. Chronic Obstructive Pulmonary Disease: Consensus Recommendations for Early Diagnosis and Treatment. *Journal of Family Practice*, S1-S8, November, 2006.

24. Steiner, S., Niessnerb, A., Zieglera, S., Richterb, B., Seidingera, D., Pleinerc, J., Penkad, M., Wolztc, M., Huberd, K., Wojtab, J., Minara, E., & C.W. Kopp. Endurance training increases the number of endothelial progenitor cells in patients with cardiovascular risk and coronary artery disease. *Atherosclerosis*, 181(2): 305-310, 2005.

Section VI

Risk Management and Safety Considerations

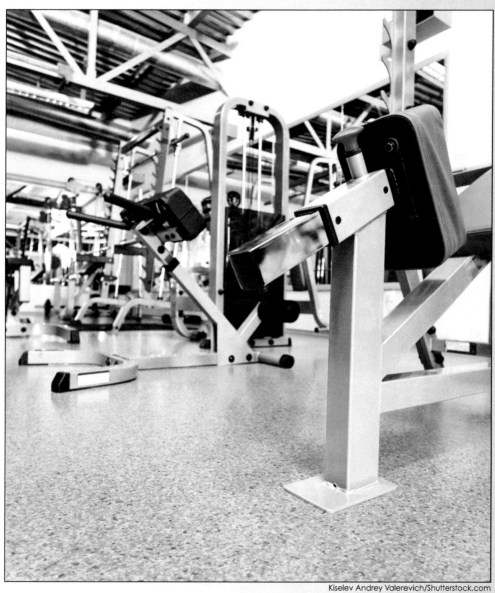

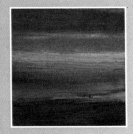

CHAPTER 25

Emergency Protocols
and Risk Management

By Stephen J. Tharrett, M.S., and

James A. Peterson, Ph.D., FACSM

Stephen Tharrett, M.S., is a thirty-year veteran of the health, fitness and sport club industry, having worked in both the commercial, non-profit and private sectors.

James A. Peterson, Ph.D., FACSM, is a sports medicine consultant who resides in Monterey, California. A fellow of the American College of Sports Medicine, he has been a contributing editor to ACSM's Health & Fitness Journal since 1997.

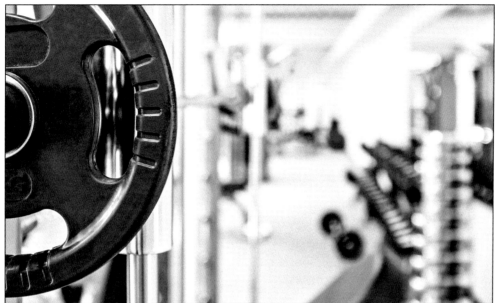

Val Thoermer/Shutterstock.com

Risk is inherent in every situation in which human activity is involved. To a degree, the level of risk for a person with a disability can be even higher, depending on the circumstances—particularly those situations that entail physical activity. As such, the primary key to dealing with risk is to anticipate it and have a specific plan for dealing with it, including doing whatever is reasonably possible to minimize it. Collectively, these steps encompass a critical process known as risk management.

Risk management refers to the policies, practices, and systems that an organization puts in place to enhance employee, member, and user safety, as well as those practices that can assist in reducing and/or eliminating the exposure of the organization to liability and financial loss due to unsafe business/operational activities. In the health/fitness facility industry, risk management applies to those practices, procedures, and systems by which an organization reduces its risk of an employee or member experiencing an event that could result in harm to the individual (employee or client) or the business itself. Among the numerous practices that play a vital role in the risk management system of every health/fitness facility that operates in a responsible manner are those protocols that specifically address the handling of emergency situations. This chapter presents an overview of the most critical risk-management practices and factors that health/fitness professionals and organizations need to understand and address in order to provide a reasonably safe physical activity environment for its employees, members, and business.

Risk Management Practices to Reduce Member/Client and Business Risk

Effectively managing the level of risk to which members are exposed is critically important to facilities for at least two reasons. First, having sound member risk-management practices can help provide a safer environment in the facility for the members, which helps reduce their chances of being injured or suffering a life threatening event. Second, properly managing the risks that members encounter in a facility can help reduce the likelihood of litigation directed to the operator that can drain the financial health of the organization. In that regard, several policies, practices, and systems exist that facilities can utilize to reduce the level of risk for their members.

Offer a Pre-Activity Screening

The first basic step in increasing member safety and reducing risk is to make sure every member and club user is extended the opportunity to complete a pre-activity screening. According to *ACSM's Health/Fitness Facility Standards and Guidelines, fourth edition,* as well as the *Medical Fitness Association's (MFA) Standards and Guidelines for Medical Facilities,* a facility must offer pre-activity screening for its users. Pre-activity screening should involve, at the minimum, screening for certain basic health risks, particularly, coronary-risk factors. Proven tools, such as the Par-Q or a simple medical history questionnaire, are extremely useful. When working with individuals who have disabilities, facilities should consider using a more comprehensive pre-activity screening tool, such as a detailed medical history that can be reviewed by a qualified healthcare professional to help identify the potential limitations of the prospective member/client.

Consider Offering a Fitness Assessment

When working with individuals who have physical disabilities, such as those that are known to limit mobility, range of motion, or cardiorespiratory capacity, facilities should consider offering some form of physical-capacity assessment. For example, if individuals indicate that they have spinal stenosis, then performing an assessment to identify the limitations of the condition could be beneficial for prescribing exercise movements that are safe, as well as beneficial to the individual.

Recommend Medical Clearance When Applicable

Facilities that utilize pre-activity screening tools should also have a system by which those individuals who are identified as having an increased risk due to their health profile are referred to a physician for clearance before engaging in physical activity. For individuals with known physical disabilities, it is highly recommended that information is obtained from their healthcare provider which sets forth the precautions that should be taken when prescribing exercise around the individual's physical limitations.

On the other hand, if they refuse to obtain a physician's clearance, the individual should sign an assumption of risk document or other form prepared by an attorney indicating they have decided not to obtain clearance from a physician and, as a result, are releasing the organization from any liability associated with their participation in physical-activity within the facility.

The medical release can be as simple as a one-page document that is forwarded by the facility operator to the member's physician or provided to the member to personally take to their physician for signature. The medical-release form should clearly indicate that the member has been identified as being at an increased risk of incurring an injury or health-related problem if the individual participates in a physical-activity program. By completing and signing the medical-release form, the physician is clearing the individual to participate in physical activity, with or without restriction. The release should allow physicians to provide any recommendations they may have concerning the individual's participation.

Require Signature of Either an Assumption of Risk Document or Waiver of Liability

A waiver is a legal document that requires a signature indicating that a client is aware of risks associated with their participation in physical activity within the fitness facility's programs and services, and that they knowingly accept full responsibility for their decision to participate in such activities and are releasing the facility from any and all responsibility for their participation, including events that may occur as a result of the facility's negligence. Because many legal jurisdictions do not recognize waivers, such documents may provide little-to-no protection for the facility operator in those circumstances.

An assumption of risk document is a legal form that members/users sign indicating they are aware of the risks associated with a physical-activity program and are assuming all responsibility for their decision to participate. The assumption of risk document differs from a waiver in that it does not release the facility from liability caused by the facility's own negligence. Instead, it indicates that individuals who sign the form accept responsibility for the actions and consequences that may result from their participation. Both documents should be prepared by an attorney and should address the following:

- The facility's programs and services to which the member has access
- The risks involved in engaging in physical activity, including the risk of a cardiac event or even death
- A statement that the member is aware of the risks associated with their participation in physical activity and that the facility has explained those risks thoroughly, and that the individual is willing to accept those risks
- The member's willingness to accept all responsibility for their participation in light of the information that has been provided. If a release is used, then the signatory must also indicate that this individual is releasing the club from any and all liability, including those events that may occur due to the facility's own negligence.

When state and local jurisdiction allows for their use, a waiver should be standard practice for every facility. If state and local laws do not uphold waivers, then an assumption-of-risk document should be used. Ideally, all members/clients should complete and sign a waiver form upon joining a facility. Both *ACSM's Health/Fitness Facility Standards and Guidelines,* fourth edition, and *IHRSA's Standard Facilitation Guide* indicate that waivers should be a standard practice for health/fitness facility operators. (Note: Some recent court rulings have upheld a plaintiff's right to legal action, even when a waiver has been signed.)

Have an Emergency-Response System

Having an appropriate emergency-response system is an essential factor for any facility interested in establishing a safe environment for members and employees. Health/fitness facilities must develop emergency response systems that help insure that their members have the highest reasonable level of safety. An emergency-response system should encompass several key elements, including:

- Employing local healthcare and/or medical personnel to help develop the emergency-response system that the club utilizes. Most emergency-medical services (*e.g.*, fire departments, emergency medical teams) are willing to assist a facility in developing an emergency-response program. Facilities can also pay for the services of a qualified person, such as a physician, registered nurse, or certified emergency-medical technician, to help develop their emergency action plan as part of their policies and procedures. According to the MFA, all medical-based facilities must have physician oversight, a practice that insures that a qualified medical professional assists with the development and oversight of the emergency-response system.
- A plan for major medical emergency situations, such as heart attacks, strokes, orthopedic-related injuries, accidents, etc., as well as a plan for non-medical emergencies such as fires and natural disasters
- Explicit steps or directions concerning how each emergency situation should be handled, including the response of first, second, and third responders to an emergency. The emergency-response system should specify the locations of all emergency equipment and all emergency exists.
- Publishing the fully documented plan and keeping the documents in an area that is easily accessed by the facility's staff. In addition, the emergency-response system should be reviewed with each employee on a regular basis, preferably on an annual basis.
- A physical rehearsal by every employee and/or contractor who is likely to be involved in responding to an emergency at least once annually and preferably once every quarter
- The use of an automated external defibrillator (AED) and cardiopulmonary resuscitation equipment (both of which are covered in greater detail in a later section of this chapter)
- The availability and location of first-aid kits within the club
- Identifying an on-site coordinator (the employee who is designated to direct the club's overall emergency readiness)

Provide the Proper Cautionary, Warning, and Danger Signage

Facilities can significantly reduce their level of business risk and provide a safer physical activity environment for their members by providing signage that is posted in appropriate locations throughout the facility. Signage should indicate the risks involved and include the proper cautionary steps for avoiding the risk's highlighted in the signage. The American Society for Testing and Materials (ASTM) has established Standard Specifications of Fitness Equipment and Fitness Facility Signage and Labels (F 1749-96), that provides guidance for health/fitness facilities regarding the signage that should be present in facilities. The key areas of a health/fitness facility that should have signage include:

- **Sauna, steam room, and whirlpool:** Due to exposure to high heat and humidity, these areas present an elevated risk to both healthy and at-risk users. Facilities should post signage that provides members/users with the basic warnings and information concerning those areas that can help them to reach a more-informed decision about whether to utilize these facilities and what steps they can take to reduce their risk.

- **Aquatic areas:** Most state and local health departments require certain signage be posted in the pool areas. These signage requirements are designed to protect users from exposure to risky behavior. With regard to signage for aquatic areas, facility operators should be familiar with the local, state, and federal laws and regulations to ensure that their facilities are in full compliance with all the legally required signage.

- **Fitness areas (cardiovascular, resistance circuit, and free weight areas):** Certain risks are inherent in the fitness areas of a facility, many of which facility users may not be familiar with due to a lack of information and/or misinformation about how to properly use equipment in the fitness area. This lack of proper information is one of the leading causes of member/client injury and business liability. Health and /fitness facilities should pay careful attention to providing the proper signage in these areas. Examples of signage in these areas might include recommendations, instructions, or notifications for:

  - ✔ The use of a spotter when performing certain free-weight movements, including those that involve accessory benches and equipment, such as a Smith machine or a flat bench
  - ✔ Guidance from a qualified health/fitness professional before embarking on a fitness program or using a piece of equipment with which they are unfamiliar
  - ✔ Stopping exercise if the exerciser experiences dizziness, pain, or unusual discomfort
  - ✔ Reading instructions and labels on equipment prior to use or asking for assistance
  - ✔ When a piece of equipment is out of order

Facilities should also provide perceived-exertion charts or target heart-rate charts so that members/users can monitor their level of exertion while exercising, which includes zones with hazardous conditions. Hazardous conditions signage is general signage that warns members/users of any unusual risk attendant to a particular physical condition or practice at the facility. These signs should be employed in a variety of situations, including:

- When equipment is out of order
- When floors are wet and the club wants to make its members/users aware of slippery conditions
- When a condition exists, such as damaged walking surfaces, loose impediment, or a related condition that would increase the risk of injury to a facility's members/users
- When repairs or construction are in progress, and the facility needs to warn its members/users of specific dangers or locations to avoid

Incorporate Preventative Maintenance Schedules and Audits

The majority of facility accidents, including incidents where employees and members experience temporary or permanent disability, occur on fitness equipment. Typically, these dangerous incidents occur because facility operators fail to properly install the equipment; fail to execute basic preventative maintenance procedures; fail to perform the necessary inspection of the equipment; or fail to provide proper instructions and supervision for the use of the equipment.

Implementing preventative maintenance procedures which are audited on a timely (e.g., daily, weekly, and monthly) basis is one of the best practices for facility operators. Such procedures increase member/client safety and reduce the facility management's level of business risk. Among the core practices that a facility can execute in this regard include:

- Ensuring that qualified professionals in accordance with manufacturer guidelines install equipment and a record is maintained of the installation process
- Employing cleaning and preventative maintenance checklists for all fitness equipment. Facilities should ensure that equipment is maintained on a daily, weekly, and monthly basis, and a record of those procedures is maintained on file. This procedure should include checking all bolts, cables; checking for loose parts; and cleaning surfaces, etc.
- Following the manufacturer's guidelines concerning the care of equipment. In that regard, facilities should have operator manuals on-site for each piece of equipment in the fitness area
- A documented system for monitoring equipment malfunctions, and noting the corrective steps to address problems
- Adherence to daily, weekly, and monthly schedules for cleaning all areas of the club
- Utilizing checklists for performing preventative maintenance of lights, plumbing, and HVAC. Facilities should seek the advice of professionals in their respective fields to help prepare these checklists.

The most critical factor is to have a system in place to verify compliance with the aforementioned checklists. Many facility operators employ supervisors to conduct regular audits of their maintenance procedures and practices. When audits are conducted, it is important to make sure the audit is documented, and the results are kept on file.

Implement Incident Reports

Incident reports are standard forms that a health/fitness organization should complete whenever an accident or incident occurs on facility property. For health/fitness facilities, it should be standard practice to complete an incident report every time an accident or safety-related event occurs at the club by eithter an employee or a member. The purpose of the incident report is to obtain the necessary information relating to a particular event, such as the type of incident, time of the incident, witnesses, extent of any injury resulting from the incident, response of the facility to the incident, etc. This information can be extremely important for situations involving insurance, litigation, and responding medical agencies.

Automated External Defibrillators (AEDs)

AEDs are sophisticated, computerized machines that are relatively easy to operate and enable a layperson, with minimal training, to administer a potentially lifesaving intervention to individuals who experience cardiac arrest. For an emergency situation, an AED is a device that can be employed to detect a life-threatening cardiac arrhythmia and then to administer an electrical shock that can help restore the normal sinus rhythm. AEDs represent the third step in the American Heart Association's (AHA) renowned "chain of survival" — after calling 911 and administering CPR.

As of January 2011, eleven states had passed AED legislation, as it pertains to health/fitness facilities (Arkansas, California, Illinois, Indiana, Louisiana, Michigan, Massachusetts, New Jersey, New York, Oregon, and Rhode Island). In addition to these eleven states, several local districts — Suffolk County, NY; Weston, Florida; and Montgomery Country, Maryland, — have passed legislation requiring health/fitness facilities to have AEDs. Similar legislation requiring clubs to have AEDs is also pending in Wisconsin. At the present time, only four states have legislation that accommodates unstaffed fitness facilities.

The movement toward requiring an AED in health/fitness facilities received strong support in 2007, when the American College of Sports Medicine, in the 3rd edition of *ACSM's Standards and Guidelines for Health/Fitness Facilities*, indicated that an AED must be a part of every health/fitness facility's emergency response plan. In addition to ACSM, the MFA, in its *MFA Standards and Guidelines for Medical Fitness Centers* mandates the presence of an AED in all medical fitness centers.

General Guidelines for Implementing an AED Program in a Health/Fitness Facility

According to the "American Heart Association's Automated External Defibrillator Implementation Guide," an effective AED Program should strive to deliver a shock within three to five minutes of collapse, with three minutes being optimal.

The FDA requires that a physician prescribe an AED before it can be purchased. The AHA strongly recommends a physician, who is licensed to practice medicine in the community, provide oversight for the facility's emergency system including the use of AEDs within that system. In most cases, the company from which the AED is purchased either will assist the club with identifying a physician to provide these services or will include those services with the purchase an AED.

A facility's emergency action plan and AED plan should be coordinated with the local emergency medical services (EMS) provider (the AED provider normally does this).

The AHA's Emergency Cardiac Care Committee, as well as international experts, encourage a skills review and practice sessions with the AED at least every six months. Regular practice drills every three to six months also are recommended.

The AED should be monitored and maintained to the manufacturer's specifications on a daily, weekly, and monthly basis. All results from those efforts should be recorded. Nearly all commercial AEDs provide this capability through an automated process.

All incidences involving the administration of an AED must be recorded and then reported to the physician who is providing oversight. It should be noted that the Health Insurance Portability and Protection Act (HIPPA) does not allow medically sensitive information to be released to anyone other than the medical director.

Each facility should have an AED program coordinator who is responsible for all aspects of the facility's emergency-response plan and the use of the AED.

All employees should complete a program in Basic Life Support (BLS) and AED certification from an accredited training organization. The two most recognized organizations in this regard are the American Heart Association (AHA), which offers its Heart Saver CPR/AED training and certification, and the American Red Cross, which offers separate courses in CPR, AED, and First Aid. These programs involve a minimum of four hours of direct-contact training. Given that such certification typically lasts for two years, an organization's employees should be required to complete such training on an every-other-year basis.

A facility should have at least one employee on duty at all times who is currently trained and certified in CPR/AED administration. Ideally, more than one such trained and certified employee should be on duty at all times.

Risk Management Practices to Reduce Employee and Employer Risk

A number of key practices, policies, and systems exist that health/fitness organizations should consider when managing their level of risk as it applies to their employees, and ultimately to their members.

Provide Background Checks for Employees

All employees in the health/fitness facility industry who are actively involved in providing personalized experiences can expose not only themselves, but also the facility, to considerable risk. Personal trainers, massage therapists, fitness instructors, and swim instructors work closely with individuals in a one-on-one environment, where the chance of a risk-related situation occurring exists.

Many health/fitness facility employees, such as child-care workers, swim instructors, personal trainers, and group-fitness instructors, are in even more potentially risk-vulnerable positions, because they often work closely with young adults and children, including those of the opposite gender. The key point that should be emphasized is that organizations should seriously consider having criminal background checks made on every employee who comes into personal contact with the members to ensure that no staff member has a prior record of unsavory behavior that might expose other employees, clients, or guests to harm.

Many organizations in the health/fitness facility industry conduct regular background checks for employee populations who represent the greatest risk, such as those who meet the aforementioned descriptions. It is important that if a facility performs background checks, it should make its employees aware of its practices, policies, and procedures in this regard.

Provide Drug and Alcohol Pre-Employment Testing

The use of alcohol or drugs can impair an employee's judgment, which, in turn, could ultimately expose other employees or members to harm. Drug and alcohol pre-employment testing is recommended for individuals employed in certain positions, such as those that involve the handling of dangerous equipment, working with minors, or working in a situation that involves close personal contact with members. Drug and alcohol testing can help reduce the risk of an employee being impaired while acting on behalf of the club. By law, drug and alcohol pre-employment screening cannot be conducted without the permission of the individual. Organizations must give their employees (actual and prospective) the option of whether to participate or not participate in the testing program.

Ensure That Employees Are Properly Credentialed for the Job They Are to Perform

The health/fitness club industry has several staffing roles that require specific licensing, registration, or certification, particularly in the arena of fitness instruction and personal training. Facilities can limit their risk, as well as the potential risk to members or clients, by ensuring both at the time of an individual's employment and during the course of employment that the credentials of every employee are valid and current. If an employee in a particular position requiring special education, training, registration, or licensure is found to be lacking, than that facility may be exposing itself to considerable financial risk. Among the positions in a health/fitness facility where an individual's credentials should be checked at the time of employment or contract signing and thereafter on an ongoing basis are the following:

- **Dieticians/nutritionists:** Many clubs offer nutritional counseling. A registered dietician is a professionally trained individual who is recognized as having the education and qualifications needed to counsel and prescribe a nutritional plan. If the employee or contractor is not a registered dietician, then the club is exposing itself to an increased risk of liability.
- **Personal trainers and instructors:** At the present time, no established national standard or law exists concerning the required qualifications for a personal trainer. Both the American College of Sports Medicine (ACSM), in *ACSM's Health/Fitness Facility Standards and Guidelines*, 4th edition, and IHRSA, in its *Standards Facilitation Guide: Health and Safety, Legal, and Ethical Standards for U.S. IHRSA Clubs*, indicate that it is essential that personal trainers and other exercise instructors have the appropriate level of education and credentials. Since 2006, IHRSA only recognizes those professional certifications with third-party accreditation from a nationally recognized certifying agency. Fitness instructors and personal trainers should have a basic certification from a nationally accredited program, such as those offered by ACE, ACSM, NSCA, and NASM.

Instructors and trainers who work with special populations, including persons with disabilities, should seek the appropriate certification related to their responsibilities. As of 2011, eight states have introduced legislation to compel personal trainers to be either registered or licensed.

Besides ensuring that their employees or contract laborers possesses the appropriate credentials, organizations should be aware of exactly what actions these individuals are legally permitted and/or qualified to perform. For example, a personal trainer is not qualified or legally recognized as someone who can prescribe supplements or rehabilitative exercises, perform massage, or facilitate muscle-activation techniques. Likewise, a personal trainer cannot diagnose a member's health status.

Have Policies for Handling Hazardous Chemicals and Materials

The health/fitness industry is a field in which many of its employees are exposed to materials that the Occupational Safety and Health Administration (OSHA) considers dangerous. Some positions, for example, such as housecleaners, lifeguards, maintenance staff, and fitness staff, are occasionally exposed to hazardous chemicals and materials. These chemicals and materials include items such as cleaning agents, paints, and lubricants. To comply with OSHA guidelines and reduce the level of risk involving the handling of hazardous chemicals and materials, facilities should undertake the following actions:

- Ensure that the material data sheets (MDS) for every chemical and agent used in the facility are posted in a visible location for all employees to view.
- Provide an MDS binder for all employees/contractors to review on an annual basis. Confirm that the employees have viewed the information and understand the issues, by having them sign a designated sheet.

- Store all chemicals and agents in secure locations. Make sure that these materials are stored in an area that is off-limits to members. These storage areas should have locks in order to prevent their access by unauthorized individuals. In addition, only those staff who have received training in the handling of these agents should be allowed access to these secured storage areas.
- Provide regular training in the proper handling of hazardous chemicals and materials, and provide employees with the proper protective apparel (*e.g.,* protective gloves, aprons, face masks, respirators, etc.)

Have Protocols for Managing Body Fluids

The health/fitness facility industry is a field that exposes its members and employees to various bodily fluids. Almost every individual who works in the industry can come into contact with bodily fluids, which can elicit the resultant risk of blood-borne pathogens. In fact, instructors and personal trainers frequently find themselves exposed to bodily fluids, such as sweat and blood, when working with members and clients. Too many facility operators fail to realize that even the handling of towels involves an increased risk of exposure to bodily fluids for employees and members. Among the key steps that every facility can take to minimize their risk in this area are the following:

- Provide training for employees. Make sure that employees are taught how to handle bodily fluids. OSHA provides training materials, as do many other organizations.
- Provide literature for employees regarding the handling of bodily fluids.
- Make sure employees who are handling towels, cleaning, or working with a member/client with an open wound wears gloves (surgical-style gloves).
- Have a system within the club for the disposal of items that might contain bodily fluids, such as bandages, tissues, or towels. If the facility washes the towels that are utilized in the facility, it should use bleach, which will help kill most of the pathogens that are carried in bodily fluids.
- If blood is visible, clean it immediately with bleach or similar agent, and do not let employees or contractors handle it without the proper protective apparel.

Have an Employee Safety Program

Facilities that want to reduce their level of risk involving their practices, policies, and procedures and the costs associated with those factors need to provide employee safety programs that address the key safety issues inherent in each job. Many of the costs and liabilities incurred by facilities result from not having a safety program in place that provides the proper education to employees about the risks of each job and how to prevent them. The key point in this regard is that a facility needs to establish clear safety guidelines concerning certain positions and job responsibilities — setting limits on the number of classes a group instructor can teach during the course of a week for example. One of the most essential employee-safety measures a facility can implement involves making sure that all accidents or incidents are immediately reported and well documented including the appropriate action taken to resolve with the incident.

Have the Appropriate Insurance Policies.

Facilities should maintain the appropriate types and amounts of insurance in order to minimize their level of risk in the work environment and help protect both the physical and intellectual assets of their business. Facility professionals should carry the following types of insurance:

- **General liability insurance:** Every facility should have a general liability insurance package that provides at least one million dollars in coverage per occurrence and up to three million dollars of total coverage.
- **Professional liability insurance:** Professional liability insurance is one key type of insurance that many facility operators fail to provide. Certain positions in a health/fitness facility, such as personal trainers, and group-exercise instructors should be covered by professional liability insurance. This insurance covers issues involving professional competency. Although most facilities and many professionals fail to obtain this type of insurance, they should. Several of the professional associations in the industry (*e.g.,* ACE, ACSM, NSCA, etc.) offer professional liability insurance-coverage packages, which members of those associations can purchase.
- **Worker's compensation insurance:** Facilities should consider establishing a worker's compensation program for their employees, especially if they have individuals who are performing jobs that expose them to injury and loss of work. In many states (*e.g.,* California), such a program is required.
- **Property insurance:** Although property insurance covers the physical assets of a business, this type of insurance can be another key element in managing a club's risk, particularly its risk of financial loss if something happens (damage or loss) to its property or other physical assets.
- **Business interruption insurance:** Business interruption insurance provides clubs with insurance against revenue loss due to unforeseen circumstances. For example, if a facility has to close for a month due to fire damage, this type of insurance would protect that organization's revenue stream during the time it is closed.

Be Proactive to Provide a Safe Health/Fitness Facility Environment

Health/fitness professionals should not assume that the risk inherent in any given situation will just go away if it is ignored. It won't. Having well-prepared and documented risk management and emergency protocols can help ensure that a facility's employee, members, and clients are provided with a safe physical environment, and concurrently protect the operator of the organization from undue legal and financial harm. Providing such an environment for persons with disabilities (*e.g.*, mobility, sight, sound, etc.) can involve its own set of accountable actions, including being fully compliant with all stipulations of the Americans with Disabilities Act. Facility operators also have a responsibility to take strategic steps to ensure that all staff personnel have a basic understanding of the needs and challenges that people with disabilities can face and act accordingly when designing and implementing physical activity programs.

SUGGESTED REFERENCES

1. American Heart Associations Automated External Defibrillation Implementation Guide. 2004

2. American Heart Association's Guidelines for CPR and ECC. 2010.

3. Fitness Management, 3rd Edition. 2012. Stephen Tharrett and James A. Peterson. Healthy Learning.

4. ACSM's Health/Fitness Facility Standards and Guidelines, 4th Edition, 2012. Human Kinetics.

5. Risk Management for Health/Fitness Professionals: Legal Issues and Strategies. 2009. Joann M. Eickoff-Shemek, David L. Herbert, Daniel P. Connaugton. Wolters Kluwer/Lippincott Williams & Wilkins

6. Medical Fitness Association's Standards & Guidelines for Medical Fitness Center Facilities, 2009, Healthy Learning

APPENDIX A

People First Language —
Describing People with Disabilities

Who are People with Disabilities?

People with disabilities are — first and foremost, people — people who have individual abilities, interests and needs. For the most part, they are ordinary individuals seeking to live ordinary lives. People with disabilities are moms, dads, sons, daughters, sisters, brothers, friends, neighbors, coworkers, students and teachers. About 54 million Americans — one out of every five individuals — have a disability. Their contributions enrich our communities and society as they live, work and share their lives.

Changing Images Presented

Historically, people with disabilities have been regarded as individuals to be pitied, feared or ignored. They have been portrayed as helpless victims, repulsive adversaries, heroic individuals overcoming tragedy, and charity cases who must depend on others for their wellbeing and care. Media coverage frequently focused on heartwarming features and inspirational stories that reinforced stereotypes, patronized and underestimated individuals' capabilities.

Much has changed lately. New laws, disability activism and expanded coverage of disability issues have altered public awareness and knowledge, eliminating the worst stereotypes and misrepresentations. Still, old attitudes, experiences and stereotypes die hard.

People with disabilities continue to seek accurate portrayals that present a respectful, positive view of individuals as active participants of society, in regular social, work and home environments. Additionally, people with disabilities are focusing attention on tough issues that affect quality of life, such as accessible transportation, housing, affordable health care, employment opportunities and discrimination.

Eliminating Stereotypes — Words Matter!

Every individual regardless of sex, age, race or ability deserves to be treated with dignity and respect. As part of the effort to end discrimination and segregation — in employment, education and our communities at large — it's important to eliminate prejudicial language.

Like other minorities, the disability community has developed preferred terminology — People First Language. *More than* fad or political correctness, People First Language is an objective way of acknowledging, communicating and reporting on disabilities. It eliminates generalizations, assumptions and stereotypes by focusing on the person rather than the disability.

As the term implies, People First Language refers to the individual first and the disability second. It's the difference in saying the autistic and a child with autism. (See the following.) While some people may not use preferred terminology, it's important you don't repeat negative terms that stereotype, devalue or discriminate, just as you'd avoid racial slurs and say women instead of gals.

Equally important, ask yourself if the disability is even relevant and needs to be mentioned when referring to individuals, in the same way racial identification is being eliminated from news stories when it is not significant.

What Should You Say?

Be sensitive when choosing the words you use. Here are a few guidelines on appropriate language.

- Recognize that people with disabilities are ordinary people with common goals for a home, a job and a family. Talk about people in ordinary terms.
- Never equate a person with a disability — such as referring to someone as retarded, an epileptic or quadriplegic. These labels are simply medical diagnosis. Use People First Language to tell what a person HAS, not what a person IS.
- Emphasize abilities not limitations. For example, say a man walks with crutches, not he is crippled.
- Avoid negative words that imply tragedy, such as afflicted with, suffers, victim, prisoner and unfortunate.
- Recognize that a disability is not a challenge to be overcome, and don't say people succeed in spite of a disability. Ordinary things and accomplishments do not become extraordinary just because they are done by a person with a disability. What is extraordinary are the lengths people with disabilities have to go through and the barriers they have to overcome to do the most ordinary things.
- Use handicap to refer to a barrier created by people or the environment. Use disability to indicate a functional limitation that interferes with a person's mental, physical or sensory abilities, such as walking, talking, hearing and learning. For example, people with disabilities who use wheelchairs are handicapped by stairs.
- Do not refer to a person as bound to or confined to a wheelchair. Wheelchairs are liberating to people with disabilities because they provide mobility.
- Do not use special to mean segregated, such as separate schools or buses for people with disabilities, or to suggest a disability itself makes someone special.
- Avoid cute euphemisms such as physically challenged, inconvenienced and differently abled.
- Promote understanding, respect, dignity and positive outlooks.

"The difference between the right word and the almost right word is the difference between lightning and the lightning bug." — Mark Twain

What Do You Call People with Disabilities?

Friends, neighbors, coworkers, dad, grandma, Joe's sister, my big brother, our cousin, Mrs. Schneider, George, husband, wife, colleague, employee, boss, reporter, driver, dancer, mechanic, lawyer, judge, student, educator, home owner, renter, man, woman, adult, child, partner, participant, member, voter, citizen, amigo or any other word you would use for a person.

Examples of People First Language

SAY THIS	NOT THIS
people with disabilities	the handicapped, the disabled
people without disabilities	normal, healthy, whole or typical people
person who has a congenital disability	person with a birth defect
person who has (or has been diagnosed with)…	person afflicted with, suffers from, a victim of…
person who has Down syndrome	Downs person, mongoloid, mongol
person who has (or has been diagnosed with) autism	the autistic
person with quadriplegia, person with paraplegia, person diagnosed with a physical disability	a quadriplegic, a paraplegic
person with a physical disability	a cripple
person of short stature, little person	a dwarf, a midget
person who is unable to speak, person who uses a communication device	dumb, mute
people who are blind, person who is visually impaired	the blind
person with a learning disability	learning disabled
person diagnosed with a mental health condition	crazy, insane, psycho, mentally ill, emotionally disturbed, demented
person diagnosed with a cognitive disability or with an intellectual and developmental disability	mentally retarded, retarded, slow, idiot, moron
student who receives special education services	special ed student, special education student
person who uses a wheelchair or a mobility chair	confined to a wheelchair; wheelchair bound
accessible parking, bathrooms, etc.	handicapped parking, bathrooms, etc.

APPENDIX B

ACSM/NCHPAD Certified Inclusive Fitness Trainer KSAs

EXERCISE PHYSIOLOGY AND RELATED EXERCISE SCIENCE

1.1.1   Knowledge of changes of basic structures of bone, skeletal muscle, and connective tissue that may occur consequent to disabling conditions.

1.1.2   Knowledge of changes to cardiovascular and respiratory function that may occur consequent to a disabling condition.

1.1.3   Knowledge of changes to metabolic function that may occur consequent to a disabling condition and the effect on caloric expenditure.

1.1.4   Knowledge of changes to muscle physiology and function that may occur consequent to a disabling condition.

1.1.5   Knowledge of changes to the central nervous system that may occur consequent to a disabling condition.

1.1.6   Knowledge of abnormal curvatures of the spine.

1.1.7   Knowledge of changes to center of gravity, base of support, balance, stability, and proper spinal alignment that may occur consequent to a disabling condition.

1.1.8   Knowledge of movement patterns and biomechanical principles in walking, jogging, running, swimming, cycling, weight lifting, and carrying or moving objects in people with disabilities that may be different from people without disabilities.

1.1.9   Knowledge of acute and chronic responses to aerobic exercise and resistance training in people with disabilities that may be different from those without disabilities.

1.1.10 Knowledge of hemodynamic responses during acute exercise, including body position changes in people with disabilities that may be different than people without disabilities.

1.1.11 Knowledge of changes to the peripheral nervous system that can occur consequent to a disabling condition.

1.1.12 Knowledge of issues related to body composition and disability.

1.1.13 Knowledge of the common secondary conditions (e.g., bowl and bladder control, epilepsy, spasticity, contractures) associated with disabilities that may affect physiological responses to acute and chronic exercise.

1.1.14 Knowledge of changes to muscle tone and flexibility in people with disabilities that may be different from people without disabilities.

1.1.15 Knowledge of how alternate movement patterns, such as upper body exercise, can impact the physiological responses to exercise.

1.1.16 Knowledge of how disability can change thermoregulation.

HEALTH APPRAISAL, FITNESS AND CLINICAL EXERCISE TESTING

1.3.1   Knowledge of relative and absolute contraindications to exercise testing and/or participation related to neuromuscular, musculoskeletal, and cognitive disabilities

1.3.2   Knowledge of the limitations of informed consent for people with cognitive disabilities prior to exercise testing

1.3.3   Knowledge of the limitations of a medical clearance prior to exercise testing

1.3.4   Knowledge of potential limitations to using various body composition and assessment techniques (i.e. air displacement, plethysmography, hydrostatic weighing, Bod Pod, bioelectrical impedance)

1.3.5   Knowledge of body mass index and its potential lack of relevance in assessing people with disabilities

1.3.6   Knowledge of alternate forms of communication for informed consent (i.e. those with cognitive, visual, and hearing impairments)

1.3.7   Ability to recognize appropriateness and use alternate forms of communication for instructing use of exercise equipment

1.3.8   Knowledge of alternate methods and adaptations to standard pre-exercise and field testing and assessment (i.e. 12-minute wheel)

1.3.9   Knowledge of the negative psychological effects of exercise testing

1.3.10   Knowledge of the lack of relevance of pre-exercise testing and assessment results in people with disabilities

1.3.11   Knowledge of potential daily variances in exercise testing results based on characteristics of certain cognitive, mobility, and neurological impairments

1.3.12   Knowledge of specific aspects of health conditions and disabilities that may affect activity and exercise performance (i.e. impaired balance and/or grip, fatigue, pain)

1.3.13   Ability to understand the purpose of and procedures for modified pre-activity fitness testing and assessment, including cardiovascular fitness, muscular strength, muscular endurance and flexibility, and body composition

1.3.14   Knowledge of additional reasons, other than traditional criteria, to terminate an exercise test

EXERCISE PRESCRIPTION AND PROGRAMMING

1.7.1   Knowledge of how to modify exercise programming based on the functional and cognitive ability level.

1.7.2   Knowledge of and ability to implement adaptive devices to assist in exercise programs for individuals with physical disabilities (i.e. grip, limb loss, joint contracture/tone, hemiparisis, paraplegia, tetraplegia, spasticity)

1.7.3   Knowledge of exercise precautions and cardiovascular considerations for specific physical and cognitive disabilities and ability to describe modifications needed in exercise prescription

1.7.4   Knowledge of valid assessment skills for individuals with disabilities in order to develop an exercise program

1.7.5   Knowledge of and ability to recognize exercises that would be contraindicated for certain physical and cognitive disabilities

1.7.6   Knowledge of the importance and ability to perform basic fitness evaluations to assess change in fitness levels or functional status

1.7.7   Skill to teach and demonstrate an adaptive exercise in resistance and cardiovascular training

1.7.8   Skill to teach and demonstrate proper posture for individuals with neuromuscular deficiencies and ability to adapt program when necessary

1.7.9   Skill to teach and demonstrate proper Passive Range of Motion Exercises for those with Range of Motion Limits and Contracted limbs

1.7.10   Knowledge and ability to apply methods to monitor exercise intensity for individuals with impaired heart rate responses to exercise

1.7.11   Knowledge of neuromuscular impairment level for Spinal Cord Injuries including differences between complete and incomplete injuries and how it would impact exercise prescription

1.7.12   Knowledge of commercial accessible fitness equipment options in health and fitness industry including accessible ergometers, stairsteppers, wheelchair rollers, ellipticals, bikes, strength equipment

1.7.13   Knowledge of the physiological response and efficiency of upper body aerobic exercise versus lower body aerobic exercise, including differences in heart rate response, submaximal workload and endurance

1.7.14   Knowledge of the diminished venous Muscle Pump in the lower extremity for those with certain neuromuscular disabilities and the effect on aerobic performance

1.7.15   Knowledge of the movement science behind wheelchair propulsion including the muscles involved and ability to create exercise programs to prevent injury and overuse in these muscle groups

1.7.16   Ability to explain and implement exercise prescription and exercise guidelines

1.7.17   Knowledge on how to adapt existing equipment to adjust to disability groups

SAFETY, INJURY PREVENTION, AND EMERGENCY PROCEDURES

1.10.1   Knowledge of the environmental effects of temperature, humidity, and pollution on the physiological response to exercise and contraindications for exercise.

1.10.2   Knowledge of the factors which contribute to skin breakdown

1.10.3   Knowledge of neurological deficits and the secondary conditions which may occur during exercise; the implications of these responses, and what the trainer's response should be if they occur

1.10.4   Knowledge of the steps necessary to prevent thermal injury

1.10.5   Knowledge of and ability to identify and react to medical emergencies specific to exercise programming

1.10.6   Knowledge of common causes of overuse injuries and how to prevent them

1.10.7   Knowledge of various assistive devices and the ability to modify (exercise) equipment to accommodate to accommodate the client's use (i.e., Velcro gloves for assistance in maintaining a safe grip)

1.10.8   Knowledge of transfers, specifically the types of situations in which transfers will be needed

1.10.9   Knowledge of the level of supervision necessary for clients

1.10.10   Knowledge of unique neurological abnormalities (e.g., spasticity)

1.10.11   Ability to position clients appropriately on equipment and mats.

1.10.12   Knowledge of the contraindication of specific anatomical positions and/or exercises.

HUMAN BEHAVIOR AND COUNSELING (persons with sensory, mobility, cognitive and psychiatric disabilities)

1.9.1 Knowledge of fundamentals of behavior management
1.9.2 Ability to apply positive principles of behavior management when providing individual instruction
1.9.3 Skills in modifying behavior management interventions based on individual need
1.9.4 Ability to use strategies that will enhance learning and mastery of specific exercise technique(s).
1.9.5 Knowledge of distinction between intellectual, cognitive disabilities & learning disabilities
1.9.6 Knowledge of impact of cognitive & psychiatric disabilities on ability to understand, communicate, learn, and master skills
1.9.7 Knowledge of myths surrounding mental illness
1.9.8 Knowledge of the ranges of hearing and vision loss
1.9.9 Knowledge of the impact of hearing and visual disabilities on ability to understand, communicate, learn, and master skills
1.9.10 Ability to identify and use alternative communication strategies for persons with hearing and vision loss/sensory disabilities
1.9.11 Knowledge of behaviors associated with intellectual disabilities
1.9.12 Knowledge of impact of intellectual disabilities on ability to communicate, understand, learn and master skills
1.9.13 Ability to reinforce and encourage appropriate social behavior

CLINICAL AND MEDICAL CONSIDERATIONS

1.12.1 Knowledge of the special considerations regarding the physiological response(s) of clients with sensory, cognitive, and/or mobility impairments and what conditions may require (medical) consultation before testing or training
1.12.2 Knowledge of common drugs for each classification (e.g. antispasmodics, colon, urinary, antipsychotics, botox, muscle relaxants) and their corresponding side effects and associated drug interaction
1.12.3 Knowledge of pain management and how to identify differences between chronic versus acute onset (i.e. phantom limb pain)
1.12.4 Knowledge of the fatigue associated with specific conditions (e.g. multiple sclerosis) and the potential triggers
1.12.5 Knowledge of the function of the inner ear, it's relation to the condition of vertigo, and it's effect on balance
1.12.6 Knowledge of assistive devices (e.g.vagal nerve stimulator, prosthetics)
1.12.7 Knowledge of the definition of an exacerbation and the ability to identify potential triggers.
1.12.8 Knowledge of the common drugs for each classification (e.g. antispasmodics, colon, urinary, antipsychotics, botox, muscle relaxants) and their side effects and associated drug interactions.

ADA & FACILITY DESIGN

1.13.1 Knowledge of the purpose of the Americans With Disabilities Act, (ADA) and general requirements

1.13.2 Knowledge of key ADA Standards related to customer service in the fitness environment

1.13.3 Ability to apply specific ADA Guidelines and Standards related to access of fitness facilities

1.13.4 Knowledge of key resources that provide information on the ADA Guidelines and Standards

1.13.5 Knowledge of other relevant disability rights laws applicable to fitness environments

1.13.6 Knowledge of the principles of Universal Design

1.13.7 Ability to identify strength and cardiovascular equipment that meets the principles of universal design

DISABILITY AWARENESS

1.14.1 Knowledge of the common disability definitions as defined in Americans with Disabilities Act (ADA).

1.14.2 Knowledge of epidemiology of common disabilities.

1.14.3 Knowledge of the negative impact of using disability labels that foster stereotyping and focus attention on the disability rather than the abilities of an individual.

1.14.4 Knowledge of appropriate etiquette when communicating, offering assistance, or inquiring about specific needs

1.14.5 Knowledge of and ability to understand the impact that disabilities have on physical, motor, social, and cognitive development

1.14.6 Knowledge of how an individual's disability interacts with the environment and how the impact of a disability can be either enhanced or hindered by the constraints of the environment.

1.14.7 Knowledge of the differences between medical and functional disability classification systems.

1.14.8 Knowledge of the benefits people with disabilities can derive from exercise and physical activity.

1.14.9 Knowledge of the barriers (e.g., physical, social, emotional, and environmental) that prevent full inclusion in exercise and physical activity programs.

1.14.10 Knowledge of the standard operating procedures used to refer clients for additional services and/or assessment that fall outside the scope of practice of the trainer.

1.14.11 Knowledge of the common support mechanisms (e.g., transportation services) available to people with disabilities in their communities that can be used to facilitate participation in exercise and physical activity programs.

1.14.12 Knowledge of resources available to keep up-to-date on best practices related to addressing the exercise and physical activity needs of people with disabilities.

Made in the USA
Coppell, TX
29 March 2021